.8 17

The Discovery and Significance
of the Blood Groups

ALSO BY MARION REID

Antigens and Antibodies with Christine Lomas-Francis
New York: SBB Books, 2008

Blood Group Antigen FactsBook with Christine Lomas-Francis
San Diego: Academic Press, 2003

Molecular Protocols in Transfusion Medicine
with Gregory A. Denomme and Maria Rios
New York: Academic Press, 2000

Red Cell Transfusion: A Practical Guide with Sandra J. Nance
Totowa, NJ: Humana Press, 1998

A Handbook of Clinical and Laboratory Practice in the Transfusion of Red Cells
with Laurance Marsh, Mercy Kuriyan and Nicolas J. Marsh
Moneta, VA: Moneta Medical Press, 1993

ALSO BY IAN SHINE

Serendipity in St Helena: a genetical and medical study of an isolated community
Oxford: Pergamon Press, 1970

Thomas Hunt Morgan: Pioneer of Genetics with Sylvia Wrobel.
Lexington: University of Kentucky Press, 1980

遗传学的先驱摩尔根评传
Beijing: 商务印书馆, 1993
(Chinese Translation of *Thomas Hunt Morgan*)

摩尔根传: 1866-1945
Shanghai: 复旦大学出版, 1986
(Chinese Translation of *Thomas Hunt Morgan*)

モーガン: 遺伝学のパイオニア
Tokyo: サイエンス社, 1981
(Japanese Translation of *Thomas Hunt Morgan*)

Hidden Letters with Deborah Slier
New York: Star Bright Books, 2008

*Der letzte Sommer des Philip Slier : Briefe aus dem Lager Molengoot:
April - September 1942*
Berlin: Osburg Verlag, 2009
(German Translation of *Hidden Letters*)

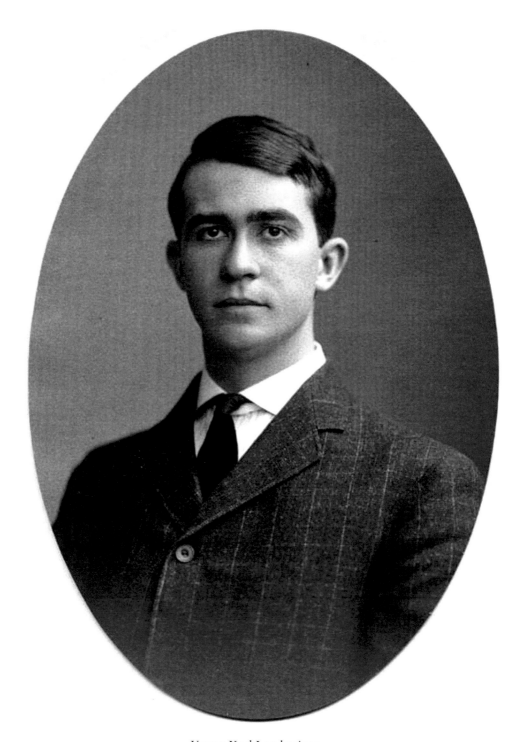

Young Karl Landsteiner

The Discovery and Significance
of the Blood Groups

Marion Reid & Ian Shine

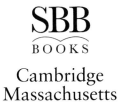

SBB
BOOKS

Cambridge
Massachusetts

Published in the United States of America by SBB Books Inc., Cambridge, MA.
SBB Books is an imprint of Star Bright Books, Inc.
The name SBB Books and the SBB Books logo are registered trademarks of Star Bright Books, Inc.

Please visit www.bloodgroups.info/ and www.sbbpocketbook.com

ISBN 978-1-59572-422-9

Designed by Catherine Hnatov
Additional design by Jiyoung Ahn
Edited by Jenefer Coates

Printed in the United States of America at Bang Printing, Brainerd, MN

        Library of Congress Cataloging-in-Publication Data

Reid, Marion E.
The discovery and significance of the blood groups / by Marion Reid & Ian Shine.
     p. ; cm.
 Includes bibliographical references and index.
 ISBN 978-1-59572-422-9 (hardcover : alk. paper)
 I. Shine, Ian. II. Title.
 [DNLM: 1. Blood Group Antigens--history. 2. Blood Group Antigens--physiology. 3. Blood Group Antigens--therapeutic use. 4. Hematologic Tests--history. 5. History, 20th Century. WH 11.1]

 612.1'1825--dc23
                    2011047142

Contents

List of Figures

List of Tables

Acknowledgements

We have received a great deal of help from many people to whom we offer heart-felt gratitude. It is quite possible that we have forgotten others, we hope they will allow the cause to be approaching senility, not ingratitude.

We are deeply grateful to the following for their insights, comments and assistance: Anthony Barnie-Adshead, Mall Blumfeld, Walter Gratzer, Peggy Hempstead, John Howieson, Pauline Marshall, Barbara Merritt, Marianne Merritt, Steve Pierce, Robert Ratner, Mark Sherman, Anna Shine. We are especially indebted to Kathy O'Herir and Christine Lomas-Francis, and Jiyoung Ahn. And Jenny Coates covered the ginger bread with delicious icing, having expertly kneaded the dough.

Interviews
Olga Blumenfeld, Shirley Busch, Gail Coghlan, Robin Coombs, Edward Einhorn, Ronald Finn, E. B. Ford, George Garratty, Eloise Giblett, John Gorman, Manny Hackel, Peter Hodges, Nevin Hughes-Jones, Lyn Konugres, Cyril Levene, Marion Lewis, Mary Lyon, Vincent Marchesi, Sandy McGreggor, Patrick Mollison, Joseph Needham, William Pollack, Colvin Redman, Laima Sauais, Wladyslaw Socha, Marjory Stroup, Patricia Tippett, Margaret Treacy, James Vogel, Mary Walker, Laura Wedock.

Librarians
Hilda Borizt, Johanna Hopkins, Bertha Ihnat, Shannon Bowen Maier, Barbara Niss, Arlene Shaner.

Institutions
American Historical Museum, American Philosophical Society Library, Rockefeller Archives, Sleepy Hollow, American Natural History Museum, Hawaii Health Sciences Library, New York Academy of Medicine, Ohio State University Archives, Royal Society, South African National Blood Service, University of Wyoming, American Heritage Center, Wellcome Historical Museum Library.

Introduction

At the American Society of Hematology meeting in 2001, one of us—Marion Reid—presented a lecture on the relationship between blood groups and disease. The talk received ecstatic applause and stunned one member of the audience—Ian Shine—who approached the speaker saying that most of the material was not known, at least to him, and as there were no books that covered the history and significance of the blood groups, why not write one? She suggested that we should write one together. This book is the result. It has been a very pleasant journey. We hope the pleasure rubs off with everyone being amazed that the thirty blood groups—that seem to be just the red cell's equivalent of the inherited moles and freckles that distinguish one face from another—are indeed the keys to life.

This book describes the blood groups anatomy, function, nomenclature, history and significance. We interviewed many of the important researchers which has enabled us to profile the personalities of the discoverers and the processes of the discoveries.

The first blood groups were discovered in 1900 by a 32-year-old Austrian pathologist, Karl Landsteiner. He called them A, and B, and C. Between 1927 and 1939, Landsteiner, now at the Rockefeller Institute in New York, discovered five more blood group antigens and in 1940, together with Alexander Wiener, he discovered Rh, named after the rhesus monkey whose red cells they had used as antigens. Landsteiner was awarded the Nobel Prize for Medicine in 1930 but thought it undeserved as he considered blood groups of little importance. The "father of immuno-hematology" did not see his work as a thunderclap heralding a storm of scientific and medical discoveries.

Landsteiner himself was a man of few words. He announced his discovery of blood group ABO in 1900 in one sentence, and his discovery of Rh in 1940 in 18 lines.

The discovery of hemolytic disease of the newborn (HDN) is as remarkable as any in the annals of medical science. Many of the figures in this story are modest, self-effacing and generous. One was a rogue, nonetheless contributed to the transformation of a commonplace and dreadful disease into a comparative rarity within 30 years of its first definition by Ferguson in 1931.

Until recently, no one expected that human beings would be better than the nematode worm as a tool to elucidate genetics. In the 1950s most geneticists in the United States, content with worms, flies and peas, opposed the formation of a society and a journal of human genetics. Today the investigation of the blood groups has elucidated the way genes are expressed, altered and silenced, and genetic blood group typing done on small blood or DNA samples can be used as calipers to measure evolution. As all vertebrates (except one arctic fish) contain red blood cells it is possible to determine where, when and how the various groups arose.

Blood groups are useful in diagnosis, in therapy and occasionally in prognosis. The simple antiglobulin test can diagnose HDN, autoimmune hemolytic anemia (AIHA), and transfusion reactions. Rh phenotyping can assist in the differential diagnosis of stomatocytosis and anemia. Elliptocytes and acanthocytes: are associated with Ge_{null} and the McLeod syndrome. The ABO and Lewis types can help diagnose LADII, which manifests as recurrent infections. The persistent infections of chronic granulomatous disease, on the other hand, may be part of the McLeod syndrome, a diagnosis that the detection of Kx type can resolve. Cataracts may be attributable to I type. Some de novo antigens may be exposed in malignant tumors, for example, T and Tn in breast carcinomas.

At the cellular level, blood groups have helped to unravel the pathophysiology of malaria, peptic ulcers, neuropathies, nephropathies, urinary tract infections, cataracts, and HDN, and they have also uncovered the structure and multiple functions of the cell membrane. Blood groups have revealed how cells communicate, adhere, move, metastasize, and take in and pass out gasses. They are important in the control of the passage of electrolytes and water, thereby maintaining the constancy of the internal environment.

The role of blood groups in therapy is of fundamental importance—blood transfusions, for instance, benefit five million patients each year in the USA alone. Yet their role is not confined to the safety of blood transfusion or the conquest of HDN. There is hardly a speciality of medicine or surgery that has not been transformed by one blood group or another. Even infertility: in 1985, an Israeli woman who had been unable to carry to term happened to hear a news item that she immediately reported to her doctor, Cyril Levene. He in turn obtained the apheresis protocol used by Paul Ness at Johns Hopkins Hospital and duly removed the p antibody in her blood, which eventually resulted in a successful birth. Later, Levene wrote to Ness: "In Hebrew 'Ness' means 'Miracle' and plasmapheresis was indeed precisely that for this patient of ours."

As can be seen from this book's long backward glance, many miracles, have already come about through the science of blood groups. And we are waiting for many more miracles to come.

The Discovery and Significance
of the Blood Groups

Chapter 1

In the Beginning Was the ABC

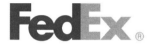

Fig. 1.1 FedEx logo with subliminal arrow designed by Linden Leader

> The Fedex arrow is not obvious until pointed out; but once seen it is not obvious why it isn't obvious sooner. The same is true for many discoveries.
>
> —Marion Reid & Ian Shine

In 1900, Karl Landsteiner discovered that there were differences in the blood taken from different presumably healthy members of his laboratory. He demonstrated that their blood could be sorted into three different groups, and he speculated that each person might eventually be shown to have their own specific blood group identity. His discoveries eventually transformed blood transfusions by providing an understanding of the failures and the successes, thereby enabling them to become progressively safer. Before Landsteiner, almost all human blood transfusions failed. One century later, risk in transfusion has become minuscule. However, the transformation was not immediate, it took many years for Landsteiner's discovery to become part of medical practice.

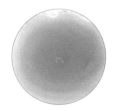

non-agglutinated red cells

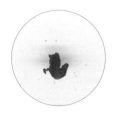

agglutinated red cells

Fig. 1.2 Red cells on slide showing agglutination

Agglutination

Landsteiner's laboratory equipment and techniques hardly changed over his lifetime [1868–1943]: he separated blood into red cells and serum, and was familiar with the agglutination of red cells (Fig.1.2) which is still an invaluable yardstick for immunologists. It had first been described by Poul Scheel in 1803, by P.L. Panum in 1863, and more clearly in 1869 by Adolf Creite, a medical student at Göttingen. Creite injected blood of different species into rabbits, and noted agglutination and lysis of injected red cells, which released hemoglobin that was excreted in the urine. When Creite removed protein from the rabbits' plasma, the agglutinating property was abolished, permitting him to conclude correctly that antibodies are protein structures that circulate in plasma, and are produced to attack foreign substances such as injected red cells, invading bacteria, viruses, and the like. Antibodies are highly specific elements of the immune response, each one combining only with its own antigen, binding many cells together to form a latticework.

Leonard Landois, working at the University of Greifswald in Germany, published a monograph on the subject of transfusion in 1875, describing in vivo and in vitro experiments on agglutination with plasma and red cells from eight different species of animals to determine whether the recipient or the donor red cells were lyzed after transfusion between different species.

Herbert Durham and Max von Gruber discovered bacterial agglutination the same year (1896) that Landsteiner[1] became Gruber's assistant; and the same year that Gruber, together with the French physician Georges Widal, described antibodies as diagnostic reagents to differentiate the diarrheal diseases due to Salmonella (typhoid) from Shigella (Shigellosis): the plasma from patients with typhoid was shown to agglutinate the bacterium Salmonella typhi. In 1899, Jules Bordet produced antibodies to red cell antigens in guinea pigs to prove that non-pathogens such as red cells as well as pathogens stimulate antibodies.

In 1900, Paul Ehrlich injected goats with blood from other goats. He found that foreign blood cells elicited a potent immune response that autologous injections did not. Landsteiner had performed many experiments in which agglutination of bacteria was the visible endpoint of a reaction, and so it was a natural extension to use the same experimental endpoint on easily accessible human red cells.

Immunological individuality

> Starting from the established fact that differences exist in the blood of different animal species, I set out to examine the question whether the individual blood differences are not present also within a species. This led to the demonstration of the individual differences, the blood groups, in humans.
>
> —Karl Landsteiner

On May 6, 1900, at the Vienna Institute of Pathological Anatomy, Landsteiner designed and carried out a simple but ingenious experiment: he took blood from himself and five of his colleagues

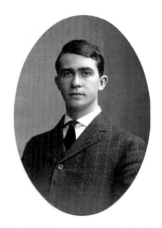

Fig. 1.3 Young Karl Landsteiner

1. From 1885–1895, Landsteiner studied medicine at the University of Vienna, which was then the mecca of medical research. He had fine teachers; Heinrich von Bamberger and Emil Fischer, Nobel Laureate for Chemistry (1902). Fischer introduced the concept that "an antibody fits an antigen as a key fits a lock." The head of the key is a small non-immunogenic antigen, whose substance and properties were discovered by Landsteiner who coined the name hapten. Landsteiner's life-long passion was to discover a chemical explanation for antibody specificity and it was for this he would have preferred the Nobel Prize, which he was in fact awarded in 1930 for discovering human blood groups. This, he said, was an accident that could have happened to anyone. He did not even tell his wife or son the day that he was notified of his Prize, "lest later they be disappointed over it." On November 8, 1930, the following answers were provided by Landsteiner to questions from a journalist: "In connection with the practical application of my blood

group studies, all I have stated is that it is possible to apply blood group tests in certain cases to prove from a blood stain that it does not contain the blood of a particular individual."

"Does the same apply also to blood group tests to prove paternity?"

"In a certain number of cases it can be shown that a particular individual cannot be the father of the child in question."

Landsteiner was not given to boasting or even to discussing his work publicly. But with colleagues, such as, Linus Pauling, for example, he enjoyed long discussions in a warm professional relationship. Aside from his work on blood groups, he investigated and clarified many current problems. He defined cold agglutinins; uncovered the pathogenesis of paroxysmal cold hemoglobinuria for which he and Julius Donath developed a laboratory test; and he demonstrated that the Forssman antigen (and some other antigens) were small specific lipid or polysaccharide molecules that together with carrier proteins (he called them schleppers) would stimulate antibody production. Landsteiner was the first to demonstrate that antibody production could be elicited by injecting inactivated bacteria.

He was also the first to introduce dark field microscopy in the study of spirochetes and showed that syphilis could be transmitted to monkeys; he demonstrated that the etiological agent of poliomyelitis was a virus that could be transmitted to monkeys by grinding up the spinal cords of children who had died from this disease and inject-

and separated the red cells from the plasma. He then mixed the red cells from each sample with plasma from every other sample. In some tubes the mixture did not change in appearance (no agglutination occurred), whereas in other tubes the mixture had agglutinated. If blood of all humans was the same, as everyone then believed, nothing should have changed on mixing. But Landsteiner observed three patterns of reactions (Table 1.1).

Tables 1.1 Males (top) & Females (bottom); Landsteiner's original data, showing results of testing red cells from apparently healthy people. It is clear that Landst. and Dr. St. were group O.

Tabelle I. betreffend das Blut sechs anscheinend gesunder Männer.

Sera	Dr. St.	Dr. Pleen.	Dr. Sturl.	Dr. Erdb.	Zar.	Landst.
Dr. St.	−	+	+	+	+	−
Dr. Plecn.	−	+	+	+	+	−
Dr. Sturl.	−	+	+	+	+	−
Dr. Erdb.	−	+	−	−	+	−
Zar.	−	+	+	+	−	−
Landst.	−	+	+	+	+	−

Blutkörperchen von:

Tabelle II, betreffend das Blut von sechs anscheinend gesunden Puerperae.

Sera	Seil.	Linsm.	Lust.	Mittelb.	Tomsch.	Graupn.
Seil.	−	−	+	−	−	+
Linsm.	+	−	+	+	+	+
Lust.	+	−	−	+	+	+
Mittelb.	−	−	+	−	−	+
Tomsch.	−	−	+	−	−	+
Graupn.	+	−	−	+	+	+

Blutkörperchen von:

No person's plasma agglutinated their own red cells. However, plasma from two colleagues agglutinated the red cells from some but not all of the others, and these he called group A; two others were agglutinated by plasma from those in group A, and these he called group B; and a third group were not agglutinated by any plasma, and these he called group C, which was later renamed O. These group names were arbitrary. He published the complete but simple experiment in 1901, but a summary footnote in 1900:

The serum of healthy people agglutinates animal blood corpuscles, but in addition, it often also agglutinates human blood from other individuals.

Emil von Dungern and Ludwik Hirszfeld assigned the names A

and B as the two "components" detected using the antibodies alpha and beta; A was the most commonly found "component" in Europe and B the less common one. The red cells that were not agglutinated by alpha or beta (that is Landsteiner's group C) they called O from the German ohne: "without". It is a good name for an amorph—a gene that is not expressed (see Chapter 3).

It is not surprising that a person with group A red cells does not have anti-A, for if they did they would agglutinate their own red cells; or that a person with group B red cells does not have anti-B. But why should anti-B occur in people with A cells, and anti-A in people with B cells? Why are these antibodies present without any obvious stimulus? The ABO groups have natural reciprocal antibodies (Fig. 1.4). Had the ABO system been like almost all of the other blood group systems that do not have natural reciprocal antibodies, Landsteiner's experiment would have failed.

Landsteiner's discovery of "the unexpected existence of clearly demonstrable differences between the bloods within one animal species" was a remarkable achievement. However, discoveries often occur before the supporting technologies exist to bring them into medical practice. The biology historian, Gunther Stent, explained that discoveries, such as Gregor Mendel's, are often not appreciated in the zig-zags of scientific progress, because the "implications cannot be connected by a series of simple logical steps to canonical or generally accepted knowledge." For two decades, Landsteiner ignored his own blood group work as well as the work on the genetics of ABO by Ludwik Hirszfeld and Felix Bernstein.

ing it into the monkeys. He did part of this work at the Pasteur Institute in Paris and part in Vienna, and it laid the foundations of our knowledge of the cause and immunology of poliomyelitis. This work was done independently by Simon Flexner and Paul Lewis.

His greatest achievements were his emphasis on chemistry as the basis of serology and the basis of immunological specificity.

Blood Group	Result of testing red cells with		Antigen(s) present on red cells	Result of testing plasma with		Antibody in plasma
	Anti-A	Anti-B		A red cells	B red cells	
O			No A or B			Anti-A and Anti-B
A			A			Anti-B
B			B			Anti-A
AB			Both A and B			None

Fig. 1.4 Reactivity of antigens and antibodies of the four major ABO groups. O are universal red cell donors, A can only be given to A (or AB) and B can only be given to B (or AB). AB are universal incompatible red cell donors (except to other AB people), but universal plasma donors.

Relevance of ABO groups to transfusion

In the closing sentence of a paper he wrote in 1901, Landsteiner remarked:

> Finally, it might be mentioned that the reported observations may assist in the explanation of various consequences of therapeutic blood transfusions.

Nevertheless, the significance of the discovery of ABO groups was not immediately recognized and was not put to practical application until a decade later. Clinicians did not appreciate the fact that transfusion reactions and even deaths were actually the result of ABO blood group differences that could be easily demonstrated by agglutination. Moreover, it took 25 years before any connection was made between maternal and fetal blood group differences and the death of a newborn from what is now called hemolytic disease of the fetus and newborn or just hemolytic disease of the newborn (HDN).

Additional ABO groups

Thus, in the beginning, based on the results of Landsteiner's experiment, blood was categorized into groups A, B, and C. In 1902, Landsteiner's colleague Adriano Sturli (one of Landsteiner's original test subjects: "Dr Sturl." in Table 1.1), working with Alfred von DeCastello (a new addition to the laboratory), discovered a fourth group, which they did not name but simply called "unspecified." It is now called group AB. Group AB red cells carry both A and B antigens, and plasma of this type contains neither anti-A nor anti-B. This AB group occurs in about three percent of the population in most countries.

Other scientists, Jan Janský (in 1907), Ludwig Hektoen (in 1907), and W.L. Moss (in 1910) independently recognized and reported the four major blood groups. Moss called them, I, II, III, and IV; Janský IV, II, III, and I. The confusion was overcome by a committee of the American Association of Immunologists who in 1927 recommended the use of A, B, O, and AB rather than Roman numerals. This terminology is still in use today. Soon after the discovery of group AB in 1902, it became apparent that group A consisted of subdivisions called A1 and A2. We now know of numerous subgroups of A and B antigens.

In the first decade of the 20th century, little was known about human inheritance and many doubted that Mendelian inheritance applied to man, while the Soviets always doubted that it applied to any animal or any plant. In 1908, Archibald Garrod gave a Croonian lecture on the inborn errors of metabolism that were Mendelian recessive diseases; and in 1908 the Royal Society of Medicine held a symposium on the application of Mendel's laws to man, at which many families with dominant traits were presented; blood groups were not included, but the same year, Reuben Ottenberg and A.A. Epstein mentioned in passing that ABO blood groups were dominantly inherited, based on two families that they tested and three they knew about. After studying 72 families in 1910, von Dungern and Hirszfeld concluded that there were two independent dominant alleles that led to the expression of the A and B antigens. In 1919, Ludwig and Hanna Hirszfeld showed that the prevalence of the four ABO groups differed between Europeans, Africans, Asians, and several other ethnic groups (Fig. 1.5). In 1924, Felix Bernstein found that the observed proportions of ABO types gave a better fit to expectation on the hypothesis of multiple dominant alleles at a single locus. It is surprising that it should have taken a quarter of a century to establish such simple major gene inheritance.

Origin of "naturally occurring" anti-A and anti-B

In 1934, M. Dupont proposed that anti-A and anti-B are not naturally occurring, but are acquired (immune); that the anti-A and anti-B must be somehow elicited. In 1959, G.F. Springer, R.E. Horton and M. Forbes experimentally confirmed this hypothesis. They compared two groups of adult White Leghorn chickens which served as suitable substitutes for humans because they have an antibody that is similar to human anti-B. For over a month while they raised one group of chicks in a germ-free environment, they raised another free range control group. The free range chicks made anti-B; the germ free chicks did not. However, when the germ free chicks were then given food containing B blood group substance, they produced anti-B, and when the free range chicks were fed bacteria with no blood group substance, their anti-B level fell (most bacteria contain B antigens, but some do not). Indeed, it is now known that many plants, seeds, beans, bacteria, and proto-

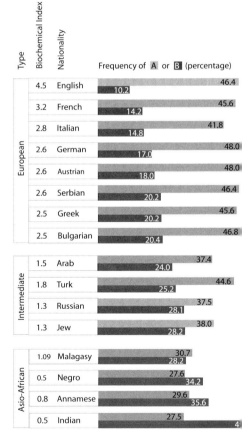

Fig. 1.5 Bar chart by Hanna Hirszfeld and Ludwik Hirszfeld (1919), shows the frequencies of A and B in 16 different populations. The biochemical index was the ratio of A (grey) to B (red)

zoa possess carbohydrate structures on their surfaces that resemble human A or B antigens; they are ubiquitous in the diet and dust to which everyone is exposed. These experiments revealed that anti-B is stimulated in response to normal microorganisms in our environment. Anti-A is produced in a similar manner.

Value of ABO blood groups

Landsteiner's discovery paved the way to defining the ABO blood groups, and within 100 years his discovery has led to five million successful blood transfusions each year in the USA alone. He could not have guessed that the number of blood group antigens would grow to 359: 317 in 30 blood group systems (as of July 2010); with 42 more yet to be allotted to a system. These antigens are encoded by over 1,200 alleles.

The discovery of ABO was the catalyst for the discovery of all the other blood groups, but before describing them, the next chapter depicts life before Landsteiner, when the patient rarely survived transfusion.

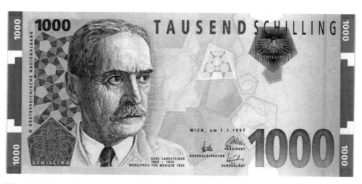

Fig. 1.6 Austria recognized Landsteiner 50 years after his death

Chapter 2

Before the Beginning

> All our progress is an unfolding, like the vegetable bud.
> You have first an instinct, then an opinion, then a knowl-
> edge.
>
> —Ralph Waldo Emerson

Plato and Aristotle considered that discoveries should be made by sitting at the feet of scholars and by reasoning, but not by experiment. Aristotle believed that women had fewer teeth than men and even though he had had two wives, he did not think to ask them to open their mouths so that he could count. The Greeks determined the distance to the moon and its size by careful observation and measurement, but that was permitted because the authorities had expressed no opinion, whereas they had decreed the number of women's teeth. The Dark Ages and the Middle Ages were characterized by an absence of observation, experiment, and of hypotheses.

It was not until the 17th century that William Harvey[1] broke away from the restrictions of Greek thinking, demonstrating by his simple experiment that blood was pumped continuously around the body by the heart in a closed circulatory system. He wrote scornfully of the Galenical belief that:

> supposes the blood to ooze through the septum of the heart
> from the right to the left ventricle by certain secret pores . . .
> But in faith no such pores can be demonstrated, neither in
> fact do any such exist.

Harvey performed his first experiment at 10 o'clock in the morning of April 17, 1616, yet he then waited 12 years before publishing his finding. It took yet many more years before his work was accepted by the medical profession and even then it had little effect on the practice of medicine. The ancient Greeks thought veins carried blood away from the heart and the arteries carried air (artery

1. Harvey demonstrated that the venous valves allowed the blood to flow only one way, thus opposing the belief that blood ebbed and flowed in the veins. He demonstrated that blood could not pass through the ventricular wall, he also estimated the stroke volume, demonstrating that the heart pumped all the blood around the body. He demonstrated that the pulse wave resembled a bag and not a bellows. For a great many years, no-one believed him; he was roundly attacked, especially in France.

from Greek *arteria*, an airpipe). The Greeks called the trachea the *trackheia arteria*, the roughened airpipe). By 1649, when there was still much skepticism that the heart pumped out blood with force, Harvey's patient, King Charles I, was beheaded in Whitehall, London. The spectators would have noted that the blood did not leak out; it squirted out in jets pumped at a pressure ten times higher than today's household water pressure.

Once Harvey's circulation of the blood was accepted—as a closed reservoir, with a recirculating pump, it was more logical to consider the possibility of transfusion. In 1906, when transfusion was less frequent than blood letting, the Canadian physician, William Osler stated that Harvey put an end to the genuflection to Aristotle, Hippocrates, Ptolemy, and Galen—for up until the 17th century it had almost become an impiety to question them. If results ran counter to Greek thinking, they were regarded with the utmost distrust. Harvey broke that tradition, he encouraged independent inquiry, direct appeal to nature, and experiment. Osler wrote that Harvey marks the break with the old tradition:

> no longer were men content with careful observation and accurate description—no longer content with finely spun theories—a great physiological problem was approached from the experimental side by a man who could weigh evidence.

While the achievements of experiment are important, perhaps Osler overstated his case: Antoine van Leeuwenhoek could still achieve wonders with careful observation and accurate description. The microscope had been invented in 1595 by Zaccharias Janssen and his son Hans, and in 1679 it was much improved by van Leeuwenhoek (Fig. 2.2), who duly wrote scores of letters to the Royal Society between 1673 and 1723 in which he described Protista (Fig. 2.3), red blood cells with a nucleus (Fig. 2.4), bacteria, sperm and the banding pattern of muscle that he observed through the lens. On 25th December, 1702, Antoine van Leeuwenhoek wrote to the Gentlemen of the Royal Society, in London:

> Here you have, very noble Sirs, the notes I took while observing duckweed and small animalcules. And while I did so, I said to myself: what large numbers of creatures there are which we do not know, and how little is that which we do know . . . Looking at the roots through the magnifnifying glass, I was amazed to see many animalcules, and those

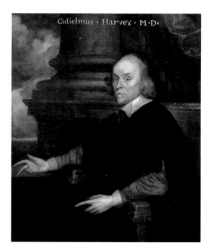

Fig. 2.1 William Harvey whose portrait in the Royal College of Physicians at Amen Corner, survived the fire of London

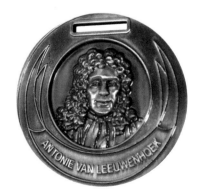

Fig. 2.2 Antoine van Leeuwenhoek South African National Blood Service Medal

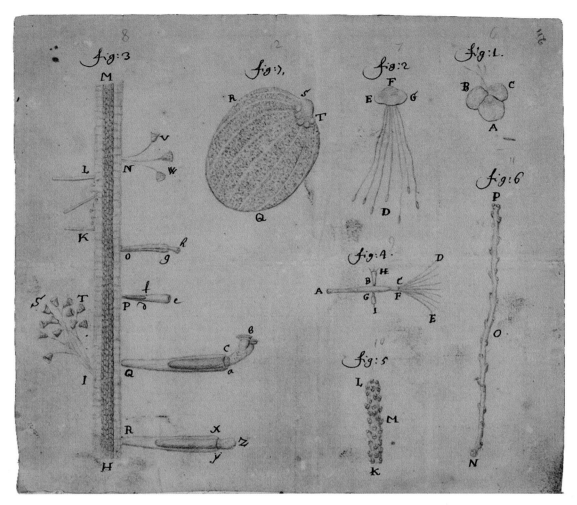

Fig. 2.3 Van Leeuwenhoek's captions below describe duckweed collected from shallow ditches and the local canal, and the "amazing animalcules" attached to it. It is drawn in red chalk by an anonymous gentleman of Delft whose exquisite detailed observations are comparable to Vermeer who was born in the same week, died in 1675 when van Leeuwenhoek became executor of his will.

Fig. 1. ABC represents a duckweed plant of a normal size . . .

Fig. 2. DEFG represents the said duckweed plant with its roots such as it floated in a glass tube filled with water, so that the roots become visible.

Fig. 3. HIKLMNOPQR represents a small part of a root of a duckweed plant such as it appeared to the draughtsman through the magnifying glass, in which roots, the vessels could be seen, with their division extending longitudinally in the roots. And when these roots (I assume) no longer serve and are as it were decaying, they become overgrown with a great many different long particles, and this mostly with small shapes that might be called flowers, as designated here in Fig. 3, partly between K and L [diatoms etc.]. On some roots I saw more than one hundred of the aforesaid animalcules, which I compared to little bells, as designated in Fig. 3 by IST [a species of Zoothamnium] and NVW [Vorticella], HIKLM in Fig. 3 with their tails attached to the root . . Now on several roots I also saw one and sometimes (but very seldom) two small tubes attached, and those of different sizes, the largest of which is here designated in Fig. 3 by RXY [rotifers].

Fig. 4. ABCDEFG represents the animalcule, [Hydra vulgaris] of which A is the abdomen, by means of which it attaches itself, and by CDE are designated eight tentacles . . .

Fig. 5. (KLM knotty protuberances;) this spectacle reminded me of the knotted threads on which so much time has been spent for some years past, and I said to myself if the ladies in our country were to see such a perfect and wonderful product, would they not have reason to regret their time and yarn spent on such useless work, which indeed does not display the least art or beauty?

Fig. 6. Part of an extended {Hydra} tentacle NOP.

of different kinds, which are invisible to the naked eye. Two of these kinds had long tails, by means of which they were attached to the roots of the duckweed plants. These animalcules [Vorticella] were shaped like a bell, with whose round opening they produced such a slight movement that the small particles in the water were set in motion thereby . . . And although I saw some twenty of these animalcules together with their long tails very quietly moving with their bodies outstretched and in an instant they contracted their bodies and tails. And as soon as their bodies and tails had been contracted, they very slowly stretched out their tails again, and thus for some time they continued to move quietly, a spectacle which I found very pleasant . . . The blood is composed of exceedingly small particles, named globules, which in most animals are red in color . . . These particles are so minute that 100 of them placed side by side would not equal the diameter of a common grain of sand . . . Thus I came to observe the blood of a cod and a salmon, which I also found to consist of hardly anything but oval figures; and however closely I tried to observe these I could not make out what parts these oval particles consisted, for it seemed to me that some of them enclosed in a small space a little round body or globule [nucleus].

Blood transfusion

A coeval of van Leeuwenhoek, and Dr Richard Lower of Oxford, transfused blood from animal to animal and animal to man, and performed the first blood transfusion at Gresham College in Bishopsgate.[2] On November 14th, 1666, two months after helping to put out the fire of London that destroyed 60 percent of the city, Samuel Pepys recorded in his diary:

Here Dr Croone[3] told me, that, at the meeting at Gresham College tonight (which it seems they now have every Wednesday again) there was a pretty experiment, of the blood of one Dogg let out (till he died) into the body of another on one side, while all his own run out on the other side. The first died upon the place, and the other very well, and likely to do well. This did give occasion to many pretty wishes, as of the blood of a Quaker to be let into an Archbishop,

Fig. 2.4 Van Leeuwenhoek's images: Red Blood Cells. "Where these oval particles lay single they had no colour, but when 3 or 4 or 3 lay on top of each other, they began to show a red colour."

2. What became The Royal Society had begun around 1645 when a group of scientists held regular Wednesday meetings. Inspired by Francis Bacon and by William Harvey, they sought knowledge through experimental investigation. The possibility of giving medicines or blood intravenously was one topic of early interest. In 1656, Christopher Wren devised two quills attached to a bladder through which he injected a number of fluids into the veins of animals: "By this Operation divers Creatures were immediately purg'd, vomited, intoxicated, kill'd, or reviv'd, according to the quality of the Liquor injected: Hence arose many new Experiments, and chiefly that of Transfusing Blood." The Royal Society of London for Promoting Natural Knowledge was granted a royal charter in 1663, with the King named as founder. The 150 fellows (it was a men only club until 1945) included King Charles II (who studied anatomy and chemistry as a hobby), Thomas Willis of the circle of Willis, Christopher Wren, John Evelyn, Robert Boyle, Robert Hooke, and Samuel Pepys. Isaac Newton was elected in 1672, and Anton van Leeuwenhoek in 1680.

3. An annual lecture series is named for Dr William Croone FRS, an anatomist.

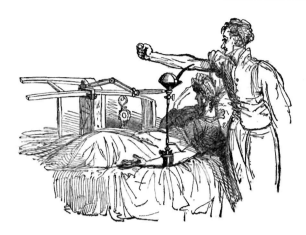

Fig. 2.5 Exchange transfusion with the Gravitator, a gravity feed apparatus, described in the Lancet in 1829

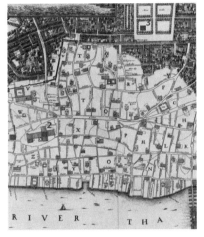

Fig. 2.6 Map of London, 1667 with the destroyed area in white. Royal College of Physicians (1), St. Paul's Cathedral (2), Bethlem Royal Hospital (3), then 400 years old, now Liverpool St. station), and Gresham College (4), now Tower 42

4. "As Christ is the lamb of God, therefore sheep's blood has symbolically become the blood of Christ."

5. A fortified wine from the Canary Islands, that Shakespeare and others called Malmsey.

and such like. But, as Dr Croone says, may, if it takes, be of mighty use to man's health, for the amending of bad blood by borrowing from a better body.

On November 23 1667, Pepys referred to the first successful human blood transfusion from a sheep into a healthy man, a 32-year-old Cambridge graduate, Arthur Coga, a doctor of divinity, whom Pepys described as "cracked a little in his head, a little frantic man whose brain was a little warm, though he speaks very reasonably and very well." Asked why he chose to have a transfusion of sheep's blood, Coga replied:

Sanguis ovis symbolicam quandam facultatem habet cum sanguine Christi, quia Christus est agnus Dei.[4]

About 8 ounces was let out, then about twelve ounces of blood from a sheep was let in, which they computed by timing, having measured the flow rate. To the procedure he made not the least complaint, not so much as a grimace. He found himself very well [probably relieved that he had not turned into a sheep, which he had feared], his pulse and appetite being better than before, his sleep good, his body as soluble [loosened] as usual, it being observed, that the same day he had three or four stools, as he used to have before. Dr Edmund King remarked that "he was merry and drank a glass or two of Canary[5] and took a pipe of tobacco, moreover three weeks later, on December 12, he had a second transfusion and was still well and survived."

When the news of the Royal Society's blood transfusions reached the French, they copied the experiments, thereby provoking hostility. In 1667, Jean-Baptiste Denis transfused the blood of three sheep and one calf into four people, two were successful, two died and one had the first recorded hemolytic transfusion reaction after his second and larger transfusion (about 500 mL):

> As this fecond Transfufion was larger, fo were the effects of it quicker and more considerable. As foon as the blood began to enter into his veins, he felt the like heat along his Arm, and under his Arm-pits which he had felt before. His pulfe rofe prefently, and foon after we obferved a plentiful fweat over all his face. His pulfe varied extremely at this inftant, and he complain'd of great pains in his Kidneys, and that he was not well in his ftomach, and that he was ready to choak unlefs they gave him his liberty.
>
> Prefently the Pipe was taken out that conveyed the blood into his veins, and whilft we were clofing the wound, he vomited store[6] of Bacon and Fat he had eaten half an hour before. He found himfelf urged to Urine, and asked to go to ftooll. He was foon made to lie down, and after two good hours ftrainings to void divers liquors, which difturbed his ftomack, he fell afleep about 10 a Clock, and flept all that night without awakening till next morning, was Thurfday, about 8 a Clock. When he awakened, he fhewed a furprifing calmnefs, and a great prefence of mind, in expreffing all the pains, and a general laffitude he felt in all his limbs. He made a great glafs full of Urine, of a colour as black, as if had been mixed with foot of chimneys.

This patient survived, and his madness was cured. Another who died was well connected; Denis[7] was accused of murder, was tried but was acquitted as the patient's wife admitted that she had given her husband arsenic. Denis gave up medicine. Blood transfusions were restricted by the French faculty of medicine, prohibited by the Chamber of Députés in Paris, and in 1679, the Pope Innocent XII issued an edict against it.[8] The practice of blood transfusion was abandoned until the nineteenth century.

The brave transfusionists

In the early 1800s, a wave of new pioneers advocated and demonstrated the therapeutic benefits of blood transfusion. In 1818, after

6. Store meant a large quantity.

7. Denis was not the first to transfuse blood, but he was probably the first to transfuse blood to man and he was about 230 years ahead of Landsteiner in recognizing that not all blood was the same: "that there are as many different complexions and various qualities in the blood, as there are Individuals in every Species." Denis was also ahead of everyone in understanding that transfusion would be useful for the treatment of hemorrhage.

He sent a report of his successful transfusion of a teenager—performed on December 19, 1666—to the Royal Society on July 22, 1667, but at that time the editor was in the Tower of London (for criticizing England's war against Holland) which delayed publication until September 23, 1667, a delay that almost lost him priority over Lower and King's successful transfusion on November 23.

Denis also reported that he had transfused 50 dogs, two of which developed hematuria.

8. The story that Pope Innocent VIII died in 1492 when transfused with the blood of three young lads rests on flimsy evidence, but as Popes are not very good at evaluating evidence, his predecessor's fate may have influenced him. The evidence that this "first transfusion" killed the three donors is more secure.

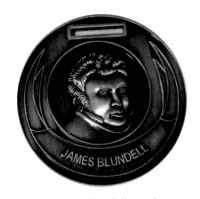

Fig. 2.7 James Blundell South African National Blood Service Medal

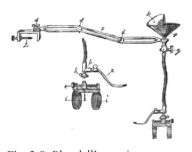

Fig. 2.8 Blundell's gravitator allowed blood to be transferred from donor to patient. It had several advantages: it obviated the need for surgical exposure of the blood vessels in the arm of both the donor and the patient. Unlike the direct connection transfusion methods, the donor's and patient's blood vessels could be used repeatedly, and the quantity of blood transfused could be measured. Blundell wrote that for a moribund patient following hemorrhage: "if instead of raising a senseless clamour against experiments and experimentors, we had only availed ourselves of the help of physiology: if we had only supplied the necessary blood: if we had only transfused [and how easily it might have been done!] at worst she could have died."

a long series of experiments with animals, James Blundell (Fig. 2.7), an English obstetrician trained at Guy's Hospital and Edinburgh, transfused women who had lost much blood at childbirth. Many died, mainly because the patients he chose were unlikely to have survived even if transfusion had been successful. Indeed, at least two of Blundell's patients were dead before transfusion was even begun! Like many of his contemporaries, Blundell felt that transfusion could have a restorative effect, even after death. Despite his initial failures, Blundell persisted and in 1825, performed his first successful transfusion to a woman with severe postpartum bleeding. Blundell connected the donor's radial artery directly to the patient's vein using a cannula of his own design. At that time, transfusions occurred with the donor and patient literally lying side-by-side. To expose the blood vessels, a cut was made in the arm of the donor and in the arm of the patient before the blood vessels could be connected. This connection was mechanically difficult and the transfusion was generally an awkward and messy affair.

Later, Blundell pioneered the transfer of blood from donor to patient using a syringe and he later devised a gravitator (Fig. 2.8), with which the mechanics of direct blood transfusion were made more practical. Blundell showed that if performed quickly enough, blood retained its restorative powers even when held briefly outside the body. In 1840, a British surgeon, Samuel Lane, after consulting with Blundell, gave a hemophiliac a blood transfusion that controlled bleeding after an operation. Blundell and Lane were the first to transfuse for physiologically sound reasons.

Direct person to person transfusions gradually cease

Due in large part to Blundell's successes, beginning in the 1860s, blood transfusion gradually re-entered medical practice.

In 1883, William Halstead (Fig. 2.9), Professor of Surgery at Johns Hopkins Hospital, who was trained by Theodor Billroth (one of Landsteiner's teachers), published a paper describing a patient near death from carbon monoxide poisoning; he removed blood, mixed it with glass beads to remove the fibrin to prevent clotting, exposed it to air, added some donor blood, and reinfused it. In 1881, he had transfused his own blood into his moribund sister following a massive postpartum hemorrhage. Both patients recovered.

In 1902 Dr. Alexis Carrel, a research fellow at the Rockefeller Institute (recruited by Simon Flexner), had developed a technique to anastomose arteries and veins that enabled him to transplant limbs, heart, kidneys and other organs for which he received a Nobel Prize in 1912. In 1908, when Adrien Lampert, the Professor of Surgery at Columbia, had a five-day-old child who was dying of hemorrhagic disease of the newborn, he had Carrel anastomose his left radial artery to the child's popliteal vein; the child stopped bleeding and recovered. This was an efficient way to transfuse blood before anticoagulation was available.

Even in the early 20th century, as the problems of blood incompatibility and anticoagulation were being overcome, doctors and patients alike believed blood transfusion was a last-ditch attempt to prolong life. It probably was, but nonetheless these early transfusions, which rarely saved the patient's life, were a necessary part of the process for it to be eventually accepted.

The first physician who mixed an aliquot of blood from a donor with blood from a patient prior to transfusion was Reuben Ottenberg at Mt. Sinai Medical Center in New York in 1910. This laboratory testing, called cross-matching, reveals incompatibility between donor and patient. Ottenberg's description of this testing was in a footnote, and he later said that if he had recognized the true value of it, he would have written a separate article. This implies that even he did not at the time fully appreciate its life-saving worth.

Prior to the beginning of World War I, few blood transfusions had been performed anywhere in the world. Sodium citrate was known to prevent clotting of small volumes of blood in test tubes or flasks. At the beginning of the war, a lower concentration of sodium citrate was shown to be adequate to prevent clotting and, more importantly, was harmless when transfused. This allowed blood to be collected and stored before transfusion, although initially storage times were rarely more than a few hours. It was soon realized that refrigeration reduced bacterial growth, thereby making it possible to increase storage time up to a few days. Numerous other modifications have since led to red cell storage for six weeks at 4°C and for 10 years at −80°C.

These innovations allowed the importance of blood transfusion to be realized during World War I. The sight of soldiers bleeding spurred on the compassionate few to save as many as possible, using stored universal group O donor blood or cross-matched blood. In the civilian sector, the improved methods of transfusion, testing, and storage had also increased the use of blood transfusions.

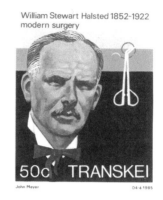

Fig. 2.9 A 1984 Transkei stamp honoring William Halstead

The increased demand for blood for transfusion was met more and more frequently from random donors rather than from the patient's family and friends. With typing and cross-matching, came the growing realization of the importance of donor selection and the phenomenon of unexplained transfusion deaths faded away. Indeed, as a result, virtually all first-time transfusions were successful.

In 1900, the discovery that blood from healthy humans differed from one another reset thinking, albeit somewhat slowly. By 1910, ABO typing and/or cross-matching had made single blood transfusions predictably successful. Many years later, after blood transfusions were given to the same patient on multiple occasions, other blood groups, were discovered. This is because the use of different donor blood increased the chance of antigen differences between patient and donor and, like immunization by a vaccine, repeated transfusions are more likely to cause the production of antibodies in the patient.

Chapter 3   In Search of Other Blood Groups

> Ask, and it shall be given you; seek, and ye shall find;
> knock, and it shall be opened unto you.
>
> —William Tyndale

As soon as Landsteiner had discovered that there were three different types of blood (groups A, B, and C) among the handful of healthy colleagues, he inferred that probably many more existed among the world's one and a half billion people. To test his hypothesis, albeit a quarter of a century later, he performed experiments designed deliberately to search for other blood group antigens.

The ABO blood groups were easy to discover because antibodies to A and B antigens are found "naturally" in plasma from individuals whose red cells lack the corresponding antigen. Moreover, observing the result of mixing plasma and red cells was a direct and easy way to test whether or not the antibody was present. Had Landsteiner tested everyone in the laboratory, he would likely have found no more than the A, B, AB, and O differences because there are almost no other "naturally occurring" antibodies associated with the other blood groups, and in the absence of an antibody, the presence of the corresponding antigen would escape detection.

Landsteiner knew that antibodies could be produced by injecting animals with bacteria or red cells from different people. He injected rabbits and guinea pigs with red cells from humans, anticipating that the animals would produce antibodies to any antigens on the red cells that were not native to the animal. For this project, Landsteiner selected 25-year-old Dr Philip Levine, a Cornell graduate who had joined Landsteiner at the Rockefeller Institute in 1925, two years after Landsteiner had been lured from the Hague by Dr Simon Flexner, the first director of the Rockefeller Institute.

Under Landsteiner's direction, Levine injected red cells from many people into rabbits. To prevent production of anti-A or anti-B, they shrewdly used group O red cells. The process was complicated by the presence of anti-species antibodies[1] in the rabbits' plasma that must be first adsorbed to allow the new antibody to be detected. After five months of patiently injecting rabbits with red cells from different people—about 10 rabbits each week—they found not one, but three new antibodies, thereby revealing three new antigens.

Discovery of M antigen

When Landsteiner and Levine tested adsorbed immune rabbit plasma against red cells from several people, they found one that agglutinated red cells from about three-quarters of the samples. This antibody detected a new antigen on the red cells. It was the first antibody to be found as a result of a deliberate search and was reported in a paper of just three paragraphs given in eleven lines of text and two tables. They referred to "the new quality which may be designated as M" but did not indicate why they chose this name.

Having produced anti-M, they wondered if, like A and B antigens, M was inherited. They tested anti-M against red cells from 286 members of 64 families and were able to demonstrate, with a little help from some friends, that M antigen showed Mendelian dominant inheritance.

Discovery of N antigen

Landsteiner and Levine encountered a second antibody, which they called anti-N. Later Levine documented that the names "M" and "N" were selected because "it was important to employ letters sufficiently removed in the alphabet from A and B, also because they appear in the word "immune".

It was clear that M and N antigens were related because of the red cell samples that were agglutinated by the anti-N, three-quarters also expressed the M antigen (were M+) while the other quarter did not express M (were M−). As depicted in Table 3.1, three different patterns were observed.

1. Anti-species is a generic term used to describe antibodies in plasma of all mammals that agglutinate or lyse red cells from all other species. The closer the relationship of animals in the phylogenetic tree, the weaker is the reactivity of the anti-species antibody. For example, anti-species in plasma from a chimpanzee weakly agglutinates red cells from a human, and vice versa. In contrast, anti-species in plasma from a rabbit reacts strongly with red cells from humans and vice versa. Thus, before plasma can be tested for a specific antibody to an antigen expressed on red cells from another species, the anti-species must be adsorbed. To remove the anti-human antibody so as to reveal the anti-new blood group antibody, plasma from an immunized animal is mixed with a sufficient volume of red cells from the species to be tested. Landsteiner and Levine mixed rabbit immune plasma with enough human red cells to attach the species antibodies present. The red cells, coated with anti-species antibodies, were then discarded. The red cells used to adsorb the species antibody must lack the antigen to which the rabbit had made a new antibody.

Table 3.1 Reaction patterns obtained by testing with anti-M and anti-N with random human blood samples

	M antigen expressed	N antigen expressed	Percent in population	RBC type
Pattern 1	Yes	No	28	M+N−
Pattern 2	Yes	Yes	50	M+N+
Pattern 3	No	Yes	22	M−N+

Relationship of M and N antigens

Details of M and N unfolded in a series of papers. The gene encoding M was named *M* and the gene encoding N was named *N*. *M* and *N* were clearly allelic, alternate versions of a gene. Levine said that neither he nor Landsteiner knew much about genetics and consulted famed geneticist Thomas Hunt Morgan and his team at Columbia University. They had proved that genes were physical entities aligned on chromosomes that behaved in accordance with Mendel's laws. Morgan, or more probably his colleague Alfred Sturtevant, advised that the M and N alleles were not dominant or recessive, but actually were co-dominant.

The apparent straightforward inheritance of M and N alleles made them popular among geneticists, anthropologists, and forensic scientists, and as markers for paternity tests. However, there was concern about the exact nature of the inheritance of M and N. Landsteiner and Levine had noticed that if plasma containing anti-N was adsorbed using N− red cells, the anti-N would eventually be removed, suggesting that the apparent M+N− red cells carried a small amount of N antigen. This opened the possibility that M and N were controlled by two different genes and that N may be a precursor to M, which was—mostly—converted to M when an M allele was present. We now know that a small amount of N is also present on GPB or a related protein.

Thus, in the late 1920s, there were eight blood groups (A_1, A_2, B, A_1B, A_2B, O, M, and N), which accounted for 18 distinct types of blood (each of the six ABO groups can be M+N−, M+N+, or M−N+; 6 x 3 = 18).

Discovery of P antigen

The rabbits that Landsteiner and Levine injected with human red cells produced a third antibody which they called anti-P, because it was the next letter in the alphabet after M and N (O having already been used). Landsteiner and Levine used this immune anti-P to test 20 families with 93 children. By so doing, they established that the P antigen is inherited as a Mendelian dominant characteristic and is not sex-linked or linked to ABO or MN types. About 80 percent of blood samples were agglutinated by anti-P, whether or not A, B, M or N antigens were expressed.

The P antigen brought the number of blood group antigens to six (A, B, O, M, N, and P). Counting ABO groups, including the subgroups of A (A_1, A_2, A_1B and A_2B), and M, N and P which today is called P1), there were 36 different possible combinations. Blood groups A_1, A_2, B, A_1B, A_2B and O could each be M+N–, M+N+, or M–N+ (6 x 3 = 18) and each of these 18 types could be P+ or P– (18 x 2 = 36). This supported Landsteiner's belief that many other antigenic differences among human bloods must exist and led him to propose:

> Perhaps if serological techniques were sufficiently delicate, every individual would have his own personal antigens in his RBCs, distinguishing him from all other individuals.

Discovery of antigens connected to MN—Hu, and He

Landsteiner made an antibody in rabbits to yet another blood group antigen in 1934, working with W.R. Strutton, and M.W. Chase. Two of twelve rabbits made an antibody that agglutinated red cells from two of 387 (0.5%) whites and 14 of 191 (7.3%) blacks. All the reactive red cells samples expressed N, and this factor was named Hunter (Hu) after Charles Hunter, the donor of the red cells used for immunizing the rabbits.

In 1953, J.N.M. Chalmers, E.W. Ikin, and A.E. Mourant reported an antibody in some absorbed immune rabbit plasma that agglutinated red cells from a small number of Nigerians and other West Africans. This new factor was called Henshaw (He), after Mr E.G.D. Henshaw, a laboratory technician in the Nigerian Medical Service whose red cells were agglutinated by the antibody. Mr Henshaw gave repeated blood donations and recruited others, including his family, to donate samples.

Deliberate searches for other antigens: Immunization of humans

Landsteiner's successful experience with immunizing rabbits and guinea pigs with red cells from humans or rhesus monkeys led him in 1928 to persuade a colleague to transfuse six volunteers with human red cells. Landsteiner reasoned that, as with his laboratory animals, it would likely take multiple exposures to the same foreign red cells to elicit production of a potent antibody. The volunteers were repeatedly injected with red cells from the same ABO-compatible donors. One of the volunteers made an antibody that reacted with about 10 percent of bloods, but it was not named.

Other antigens are found opportunistically

During the 1930s, evidence was mounting that antibodies to as yet unnamed antigens on human red cells existed. At this time, blood donors were selected by ABO group. Blood was not tested for M or N because no anti-M or anti-N had been stimulated as the result of transfusion or pregnancy. M and N antigens are not immunogenic. Alexander Wiener, and Raymond Peters wrote in 1940: "Despite the performance of hundreds of thousands of transfusions every year, in which donors are selected without regard to their M-N types, not a single hemolytic reaction can be traced to this source." Even though the recipient and donor were identical for ABO,

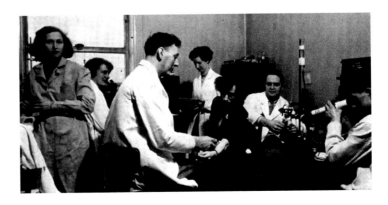

Fig. 3.1 Patrick Mollison drawing blood in his laboratory in London in 1939

occasionally the patient would have a transfusion reaction. These reactions were called "intragroup" incompatibilities. To detect these intragroup incompatibilities, some clinicians believed a pre-transfusion test between recipient and donor blood should be performed, either in vitro on a slide, or in vivo[1] by transfusing a small enough quantity of blood to cause observable lysis but not cause harm. As will be described in subsequent chapters, these incompatibilities were due to antibodies to many blood group antigens.

Most antibodies to other blood antigens are produced in a person exposed to red cells that express antigens not present on their own red cells. The immune response does just what it is designed to do—it fights off invaders. When the number of blood transfusions was relatively small, there was little chance that a new antibody would be induced. Even if a patient developed a new antibody, it would remain undetected until the patient was transfused with red cells expressing the same antigen.

Another terrible consequence of incompatibility occurs between the blood group of an unborn baby and its mother. This has long been one of the major causes of infant mortality. Until 1941, it was not known to bear any relationship to blood groups. But as the next chapter will show a series of astonishing discoveries determined that blood group incompatibility was the culprit.

1. An in vivo crossmatch involves injecting 5 to 10 mL blood into one arm; waiting five minutes and then collecting a blood sample from the other arm. The blood is centrifuged and the plasma observed for hemolysis. The test is remarkably sensitive.

Chapter 4   **Ruth Darrow's insight**

> Discovery consists in seeing what everyone has seen,
> and thinking what no one has thought.
>
> —Albert Szent-Györgyi

For giving Adam an apple, God said to Eve, "In sorrow thou shalt bring forth children," and it was so until the last century. From the Garden of Eden until Queen Victoria, the maternal mortality rate was about three percent and infant mortality ten percent. Since then, in countries with high maternal literacy, the maternal mortality rate has fallen to 1:10,000 live births. At the same time, the infant mortality rate has fallen to 0.3 percent.

The improvement in the chance of having a live healthy child is due in part to the nearly complete conquest of Rh hemolytic disease of the newborn (HDN). Formerly it was manifest as hydrops or jaundice of the newborn or congenital progressive anemia or *erythroblastosis fetalis*. Hydrops had been recognized for a long time by people who did not realize that these several different diseases of the newborn were in fact all one, something that eluded everyone until 1931 when John Ferguson unified the disease. In 1609, Louise Bourgeois, official midwife to Marie de Medici (second wife of King Henry IV of France), graphically described this devastating condition thus:

> Of a lady whom I delivered of two children after seven months: the daughter was hydropic, but the son was not . . . . She was happily delivered, without much trouble, of a girl, who came head first. As she was coming out, I felt a hardness such as reminded me of a child which M. du Laurens, first Physician to the King, said he had seen at Sens in Burgundy, at the premises of a surgeon, and which a woman bore at eighteen years of age, and it was hard as a stone. I thought I was holding a similar child. I saw a girl, alive and hydropic,

from the head to the thighs and up to the lips so hard that the child could not have been harder. It seemed as if one was touching wood. She had a fat belly, stretched like a ball, extremely black and because of the tension there was not the smallest vein in it that was unbroken. The child lived about a quarter of an hour . . . The girl's placenta was full of yellow mucus and the veins through which the nourishment was carried to her umbilical vein were full of yellow blood, like that which one normally draws from a pleuritic.

There had been many other reports of babies with hydrops or severe jaundice. In 1910, erythroblastosis was described as a separate entity, while in 1920 progressive anemia was described. In 1931, a Harvard pathologist, John Ferguson, was the first person to recognize that these were different manifestations of a "definite disease entity of the newborn" with ectopic erythropoiesis as the outstanding common feature.

Ferguson performed autopsies on six babies with erythroblastosis that died at or soon after birth; two with hydrops, three with jaundice, and one with probable bilirubin deposition in the liver. He reported his findings in 1931 in the *American Journal of Pathology*:

> Normally at birth the liver has completely ceased to function as a hematopoietic organ. . . . The marked enlargement of the liver and spleen, which in Case IV was over eleven times larger than normal for a newly born infant, and the active hematopoiesis in the bone marrow, liver, spleen and other organs, strongly suggest that these cases may be related to the 'anemias' of infancy and early childhood.

One year later, L.K. Diamond, K.D. Blackfan, and J.M. Baty, three pediatricians, also at Harvard, described pretty much what Ferguson had described the year before although they received the credit. They called the disease *erythroblastosis fetalis*; they presented 20 cases with clinical and laboratory data, two with hydrops, twelve with jaundice, and six with anemia. Autopsies were done on nine of the babies, all of whom had erythroblastosis. They attributed the disease (incorrectly) to a metabolic defect:

> The disease appears to be a disturbance of the metabolism of the hematopoietic system resulting first, in either a fail-

ure of maturation of erythrocytes or in an overgrowth of immature forms of erythrocytes, second in the delivery of immature nucleated erythrocytes in large numbers to the peripheral circulation; and third, in the increased destruction of the erythrocytes, including the nucleated forms.

In the early 1930s, Louis Diamond was one of the first to treat HDN with blood transfusion:

> We first treated newborn infants with jaundice and anemia, using compatible blood from the father (therefore Rh-positive) for transfusion. Many transfusions were often necessary since the red cells did not seem to survive long.

Ruth Renter Darrow (1895-1956)

In 1938, Ruth Darrow (Fig. 4.1), a Chicago physician, shifted the focus of attention from abnormal blood production (erythroblastosis), that she correctly termed "a symptom", to abnormal blood destruction (lysis), "the cause". She wrote a comprehensive review of HDN, based on 70 papers from G. Schmorl's description of kernicterus in 1904 to M.T. Macklin's 1937 report on the conjunction of hydrops and *icterus gravis*. It was also based on her observations of her own child who had died of HDN. She described the clinical features, the epidemiology, genetics, and pathology and reviewed the existing theories of causation: a metabolic defect in red cell production, maternal anemia, pre-eclamptic toxemia, biliary obstruction, a Mendelian recessive trait, a Mendelian dominant trait, and she found them all wanting. She proceeded to describe a cause of HDN that was consistent with its strange features, for instance that at birth the baby is often strong but soon deteriorates, especially if it is breast-fed.

Darrow's explanation was novel, consistent with all the known facts, and true. She followed the Harvard investigator's reasoning that the diverse manifestations—severe jaundice, anemia and hydrops appearing in different family members—indicated that they were parts of the same disease, generally with excess erythropoiesis. She insisted that a theory of cause and effect must account for the following clinical and epidemiological features of the disease:

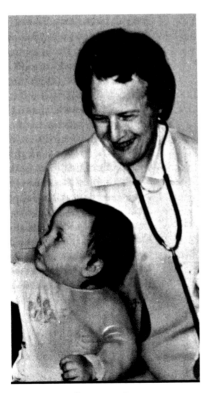

Fig. 4.1 Ruth Renter Darrow

(1) The apparent absence of any hereditary factor

(2) The fact that the birth of healthy, normal children may precede that of the child in whom the condition first manifests itself in a family

(3) The frequent familial tendency

(4) The apparent health of the parents

(5) The apparent absence of significant factors in the prenatal history in the large majority of cases

(6) The presumptive association of edema, grave jaundice and anemia of the newborn

(7) The clinical symptoms

(8) The observations at necropsy

(9) The erythroblastosis.

Darrow's insights

In 1938 Ruth Darrow gave her hypothesis of HDN:

If, now, the possible mechanisms giving rise to destruction of erythrocytes are reviewed, it is found that all may be eliminated from consideration save one, the destruction of red cells by some form of immune reaction. If the destruction of red cells by the action of specific immune bodies is tentatively considered to represent the pathological mechanism underlying this disease, one may reconstruct the etiologic events as follows: The mother is actively immunized against fetal red cells or some component of them. The immunization may conceivably occur as the result of an accident within the placenta whereby the fetal cells or their hemoglobin gain entrance to the maternal blood sinuses. The antibodies formed in the maternal organism may then pass to the child through the placenta or possibly to an even greater extent through the colostrum and milk, since the diminution of red cells in congenital anemia appears to be most acute following birth. The time elapsing before such antibodies are present in the infant in sufficient concentration to produce a marked effect may correspond to the delay in the appearance of symptoms noted in most cases of congenital anemia. Such a transfer of immune bodies from an actively immunized mother to the fetus or newborn child sets up in the offspring a state of passive immunity. Such immunity is relatively short lived and would eventually disappear completely, leaving no

trace to be passed on to a succeeding generation. Furthermore, each child born and suckled subsequent to this active
immunization in the mother would possess to a greater or
less degree a passive immunity to the specific antigen, while
any child born before the immunization of the mother would
be entirely unaffected. . . . This conception of possible events
leads to the formulation of a hypothesis which thus explains
adequately not only the familial tendency in this disease
but likewise its definite and distinctive distribution among
the children of an affected family. In the operation of such
a mechanism the mother would show no symptoms, yet she
would transmit a destructive influence to successive offspring
through the placenta and through her milk. This mechanism,
incidentally, bears no relation to a difference in blood groups
in mother and child; nor is such a difference a factor in this
group of diseases.

Ruth Darrow had brilliant insight, which was worthy of a Nobel Prize. In the history of medicine there has never been another
comparable example. Darrow's hypothesis came long before the
determination of the structure of fetal hemoglobin, or indeed any
hemoglobin. In 1938, she envisaged before Diamond, Landsteiner,
Wiener, and Levine that a maternal antibody could cause red cell
destruction in a child! Darrow had proposed that fetal red cells or
some component was likely to be immunologically different from
adult hemoglobin, that it might well gain access to the maternal
circulation, and thus actively immunize the mother. Furthermore,
she postulated that the resulting maternal antibody might cross the
placenta and destroy the fetal red cells. Darrow concluded, "An
antigen-antibody reaction seems to explain best all aspects of these
related disorders." In other words, abnormal destruction of fetal
red cells was one of the fundamental pathological processes.

The primary influence giving rise to these pathologic processes
in a series of offspring in the same family must be traced to
the mother. The placenta seems to be the means of transmission
of the destructive influence from mother to fetus.

The concept that the placenta was the means of transmission of
the destructive influence from fetus to mother to fetus was such a startling idea that it is surprising that she introduced it so casually.

Darrow considered the possibility that the blood groups were the provoking antigen but Diamond's data showed that most couples were ABO compatible; she could hardly have predicted the role of the Rh blood group before the Rh blood group had been discovered. At the time only ABO, MN and P1 blood group antigens were known, and we now know that ABO incompatibility is a rare cause of HDN and that M, N, and P1 effectively never cause HDN. In 1923, Reuben Ottenberg at Mt. Sinai Hospital had suggested that it seemed possible that several other unexplained diseases, particularly the jaundice of the newborn, and perhaps even certain cases of hemorrhagic disease of the newborn, may be due to accidental placental "transfusion" of incompatible blood. Darrow did not cite and presumably did not know of this paper[1], in which it was a passing comment.

The arcane antibody is revealed

In 1939, P. Levine and R. Stetson found the missing piece of critical evidence, the antibody that was the cause. But even with Darrow's reasoning as a beacon, it took Levine and Wiener two years to reach the same understanding. In 1980 Levine remarked:

> In my 56 years devoted to active research in the laboratory, I invariably discovered surprisingly "new" gems in reviewing the literature of the past.

One gem that Levine missed was Darrow's publication. This does not detract from Levine's revolutionary realization that the Rh antigen was the cause of HDN. Pediatrician Wolf Zuelzer recalls Levine's visit to his laboratory in Detroit in this connection, which took place sometime in 1941:

> Bubbling with excitement yet reluctant to overturn established dogma and aware that he was venturing into uncharted seas, Levine was visibly reassured when his attention was called to Ruth Darrow's paper in the Archives of Pathology. But the serological evidence [Levine's] was conclusive of itself.

1. Over the past 100 years, the methods by which we can search the literature have changed dramatically. Darrow would have searched up to four indexes each year, with the added difficulty that placental leakage was neither a recognized subject heading, nor was the disease itself indexed. When a suggestive reference was found, two searches were then required, the first for a serial number and then a second search for the articles that were serially listed giving title and author. And then one had to find the journal, read it, take handwritten notes, or write for a reprint. By contrast today, over 5,450 journals are indexed and available electronically and mostly free and the same search takes seconds. In July 2003, when interviewed, Professor Vincent Marchesi commented:

> I don't want to sound like an old fogy, but one of the problems in the daily reality of doing science nowadays is keeping track of what others have done. Never mind the "ancients," I mean people who have done things last week! There is just so much being published every week.

Chapter 5

Discovery of Rh

> In the fields of observation, chance favors only the mind
> that is prepared.
>
> —Louis Pasteur

The observation of incompatibility between a mother and her fetus was key to the opportunistic discovery of the next blood group, Rh or D. The ABO, MN, and P1 antigens, which were revealed through deliberate search, were just the beginning of the intriguing world of blood groups. Of today's 30 blood group systems, 24 were discovered because of incompatibilities during pregnancy or transfusion.

Intragroup incompatibility in a pregnant lady

From 1935, Levine worked at Beth Israel Hospital in Newark, New Jersey where he was consulted regarding a pregnancy case that would reveal the next blood group. In late July 1937, Mrs Mary Seno, a 25 year-old, was six months pregnant with her second child. She was briefly admitted to Bellevue Hospital, New York due to pre-eclamptic toxemia that, if untreated, might have progressed to epileptic-like fits, coma and death. In September, she was readmitted to Bellevue Hospital in labor. She experienced heavy bleeding and delivered a "badly decomposed" stillborn fetus weighing 1 pound 5 ounces.

Mrs Seno lost so much blood that it was deemed necessary to transfuse her. As was typical in the 1930s, she was transfused with blood from her ABO-compatible husband (Mr and Mrs Seno were both group O). Ten minutes after the transfusion was started, Mrs Seno experienced shaking, chills, and pain in her head and lips. Her urine was dark red. The transfusion was stopped. Her bleeding continued and eight cross-matched, compatible, transfusions from different donors were given. She did not react to any of them, and recovered.

In laboratory tests, the patient's plasma agglutinated red cells from her husband and from most group O donors. Of 50 blood samples tested, only eight were compatible. The obstetrical staff handling this case consulted with hematologist Rufus Stetson, an expert on blood transfusion. At a time when most doctors were concerned only with ABO compatibility for transfusion purposes, Stetson was aggressively searching for other causes of intragroup incompatibilities. He considered that ABO typing and 'simple' compatibility testing led to errors. He also suspected that there were antibodies unrelated to ABO groups. Although the immediate crisis for Mrs Seno was over, Stetson wanted to understand what had happened. In October 1937, he consulted Philip Levine.

Levine tested Mrs Seno's plasma against 54 blood samples, and found only 13 were compatible. The reactions were not due to ABO, M, N, or P1. In most cases of unexplained transfusion reactions, no antibodies or incompatibilities could be detected by the tests then available. Indeed, later in the year when another sample was collected from Mrs Seno, the direct agglutinating activity was no longer detectable. The crude test of the day, the direct agglutination test is depicted in Fig. 5.1.

Unlike most intragroup transfusion reactions, which were in patients who had been previously transfused, Mrs Seno's reaction had occurred during her first transfusion. Levine deduced that her antibody had been produced in response to an antigen associated with the fetus. At the time, he wrote:

> one may assume that the products of the disintegrating fetus were responsible not only for the toxic symptoms, but also for the iso-immunization. Presumably the immunizing property in the blood and/or tissues of the fetus must have been inherited from the father. Since this dominant property was not present in the mother, specific immunization conceivably could occur.

This provided an explanation why red cells from Mrs Seno's husband were incompatible with her plasma, and caused the transfusion reaction. When Levine and Stetson wrote up this case with their discovery of a new antigen and a hypothesis how it caused HDN, they did not name the antigen. Some have attributed that to their compliance with Landsteiner's injunction to Levine, when he left the Rockefeller

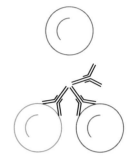

IgM antibody binds and crosslinks antigen-positive red cells causing agglutination.

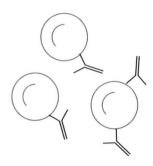

IgG antibody binds to but cannot crosslink antigen-positive red cells: no agglutination

Fig. 5.1 Schematics for direct typing of RBCs for a blood group antigen. Red cells of unknown type are mixed with, for example, anti-A and anti-B in separate tubes. After incubation, the sedimented or centrifuged red cells are observed for agglutination. The presence of agglutinates indicates that a reaction has occurred and the red cells express, that is to say possesses, the antigen detected by the antibody. The absence of agglutinates indicates the red cells do not express the antigen, or that the antibody is IgG.

Institute in 1932, not to work on blood groups. While Levine had perceived that a blood group incompatibility was the cause of fetal death, he did not see the full implications. Working in his laboratory, away from the hospital, Levine had received only part of the story. He apparently did not know why her baby had died, however ultimately he made the connection.

Intragroup incompatibility in rabbits

At the same time, Landsteiner and Alexander Wiener were immunizing rabbits in search of even more blood groups. They used red cells from rhesus monkeys because they are close relatives to humans and Landsteiner suspected that the red cells would express human antigens. After they removed unwanted anti-species antibodies by the adsorption procedure that they had used to uncover anti-M, anti-N, and anti-P1, they then found a remaining antibody that was new; it reacted weakly with about 85% of the human red cell samples. They called the antibody "anti-Rh", after the rhesus monkeys. Although most of this work was done in 1937, Wiener and Landsteiner delayed reporting their results while trying to make a stronger preparation of the new antibody. They later succeeded by immunizing guinea pigs instead of rabbits.

The manuscript written by Landsteiner and Wiener to describe anti-Rh was published one year after Levine's and consisted of merely 18 lines. A year later, Landsteiner, Wiener and Peters wrote another paper suggesting that anti-Rh could cause intragroup transfusion reactions of which Mrs Seno's transfusion reaction was an example.

Intragroup incompatibility in humans

With the possibility of intragroup incompatibility in mind, Landsteiner and Wiener accumulated cases in which transfusion reactions had occurred in ABO-compatible donor/patient pairs. By 1941, they had ten such cases. In direct testing, the plasma from these cases contained anti-Rh, further convincing Wiener that anti-Rh was related to the previously unexplained transfusion reactions. While Levine had conjectured that Mrs Seno's antibody was made in response to her dead fetus, Wiener independently concluded, based on his detailed review of cases that most such reactions occurred in people who had been transfused or pregnant. He also realized that exposure to fetal red cells through pregnancy was a likely source of immunization.

In the meantime, Levine had received a blood sample from another woman who had had a transfusion reaction after receiving blood from her husband to replace blood lost by postpartum bleeding. This sample was provided by Dr Lyman Burnham in nearby Engelwood, New Jersey. The baby of this patient had also died, but again this case was considered a blood transfusion problem. Four months later, Burnham had a similar case. The mother had a reaction following transfusion of her husband's blood. In this case, the baby was diagnosed with *erythroblastosis fetalis*, and Burnham specifically brought this diagnosis to the attention of Levine.

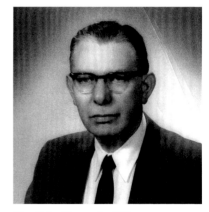

Fig. 5.2 Alexander Wiener

Levine recognized the connection. He realized that the baby's red cells (expressing paternally derived blood group antigens) crossed the placenta, and entered the mother's circulation where they stimulated her to produce antibodies. Thus sensitized, she responded strongly when transfused with her husband's blood. In addition, he recognized that the mother's antibodies also crossed the placenta, entering the fetal circulation where they destroyed the red cells. This concept was revolutionary, because at the time, despite the insight of Hirszfeld, Darrow and others, the placenta was widely thought to be a barrier preventing anything as large as a red cell passing between mother and her fetus.

Levine and co-workers published their theory in the *Journal of the American Medical Association*, March 1, 1941, just about the time Landsteiner and Wiener submitted their paper to the *Proceedings Society Experimental Biology and Medicine*. Levine found that in over 90% of *erythroblastosis fetalis* cases, the mother was Rh-negative and the father Rh-positive.

To see whether the antibody in Mrs Seno's plasma was the same as the rabbit anti-Rh, Levine and Wiener exchanged samples. It appeared that it was, and Levine referred to the antibody in Mrs Seno's plasma as anti-Rh. Unfortunately, Levine and Wiener conducted a bitter public rivalry, each claiming to be the discoverer of Rh. Both had a claim—Wiener, because he and Landsteiner had made the antibody and then shown it reacted the same as the one in humans; Levine, because his report on Mrs Seno had been published first, he demonstrated that the antibody agglutinated 80% of the population, and he had included the

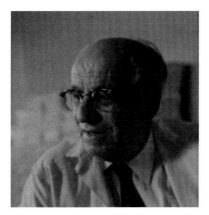

Fig. 5.3 Philip Levine

mechanism by which the antibody arose and caused both transfusion reactions and *erythroblastosis fetalis*. Their rivalry was one of the major feuds over priority in modern medical history, and almost as bitter as that of Newton and Leibniz over the discovery of calculus or that of Gallo and Montagnier over who identified HIV.

Animal and human anti-Rh are not the same

As time passed, it became apparent that human anti-Rh and animal anti-Rh were not identical. First, the red cells from all (i.e., Rh+ and Rh–) newborn babies reacted equally well with the guinea pig anti-Rh reagent. Second, tests showed that Rh– red cells (typed with human reagents) completely adsorbed the anti-Rh in the guinea pig plasma but not anti-Rh in human plasma. Third, if Rh– red cells (typed with human reagents) were injected into guinea pigs, the animals made the same antibody as when Rh+ red cells were injected. The antigen detected by the guinea pig anti-Rh was similar, but not identical to the human antibody. Later, rare human examples of Rh+ red cells (typed by human anti-Rh) were not agglutinated by the guinea pig antibody. By this time, the Rh name was strongly embedded into blood group antigen terminology, so a new one was selected for the antibody made by Landsteiner and Wiener's rabbits and guinea pigs. In 1963, at the suggestion of Levine, it was called "LW"—for Landsteiner and Wiener. Landsteiner had died and Wiener was not pleased with the name. Until his death, Wiener vehemently, although incorrectly, believed that his rabbits and guinea pigs indeed made anti-Rh and not anti-LW, maybe because if the animals made anti-LW, he would have no claim to Rh priority.

Clinical relevance of Rh

The discovery of Rh was of major importance in transfusion therapy because it provided the way to avoid Rh incompatible transfusions. After the discovery of Rh, many other antibodies against blood group antigens were found. However, before describing them, we will discuss the next developments in Rh HDN.

Chapter 6

Rh HDN: Treatment and Prevention

Steps to the acceptance of a scientific theory
i)   This is worthless nonsense.
ii) This is an interesting, but perverse, point of view.
iii) This is true, but quite unimportant.
iv) I always said so.

—J.B.S. Haldane

The Oxford Textbook of Medicine lists about two thousand diseases, of which very few are both treatable and preventable. Rh hemolytic disease of the newborn (HDN) stands out because it defied definition for many centuries, yet within a third of a century after Ferguson had brought together four diverse manifestations into one disease, the etiology was identified, the pathology was elucidated, the treatment was developed, and a method of prevention was validated.

For millennia, HDN was a major cause of intrauterine deaths, neonatal deaths, and brain damage. Today the disease is on its way to extinction; indeed many physicians have never personally observed its devastations.

To understand, treat, and prevent a disease within 33 years of its identification is a feat unequaled in the history of medicine. Yet perhaps the reason this great achievement failed to receive the notice it deserved was that blood groups occupy a secondary place in medical thinking, receiving skimpy attention in almost all medical textbooks (*Nathan and Oski's Hematology of Infancy and Childhood* being a dazzling exception). Even the Nobel committee dozed off, missing the opportunity to hand out prizes to some of the worthy researchers who appear in this chapter.

Pathophysiology

Between 1931 and 1958, the etiology of HDN was recognized to involve the following elements:

- The Rh antigen.
- The Rh-negative mother lacks the Rh antigen that her child inherited from the father.
- The child's Rh-positive red cells pass through the placenta into the maternal circulation[1] at delivery, and to a lesser extent, throughout pregnancy.
- The mother's B lymphocytes produce an antibody, immunoglobulin G (IgG), against the child's Rh antigen.
- Antibody production is primed at the first exposure; and at the next pregnancy with an Rh-positive child, large quantities of antibodies are produced.
- The mother's Rh IgG antibodies enter the child's circulation from the mother's milk or by passing across the placenta.
- Once in the fetal circulation, the antibodies attach to the fetal red cells, leading to their destruction.
- Red cell destruction causes anemia, which stimulates increased red cell production and releases erythroblasts into the circulation.
- Lysis releases hemoglobin that is converted to bilirubin that is transported into liver cells where it binds to ligandin, whose concentration is low at birth. It is conjugated with glucuronic acid to a water-soluble form in the endoplasmic reticulum.
- The liver is the main site of erythropoiesis until the 24th fetal week. Production ceases soon after birth, except in HDN, when most of the liver can be devoted to erythropoiesis, which impairs the liver's ability to conjugate bilirubin and synthesize albumin. Anemia and heart failure impair liver function.
- When the concentration of unconjugated bilirubin exceeds 18mg/dL, it binds to the neurons in the base of the brain causing kernicterus.
- Some babies develop hydrops. This is attributable to low plasma albumin reducing plasma osmotic pressure, to increased central venous pressure, increased capillary permeability, heart failure, and increased levels of atrial natriuretic peptide.

1. History of placental leakage

Around 1750, William and John Hunter demonstrated that wax would not pass from the maternal into the fetal circulation, confirming the placenta as an impermeable barrier. The first clue that the barrier might be incomplete came in 1902 from Simon Flexner (the Louisville KY pathologist who was director of the Rockefeller Institute from 1901-1935, and recruited Landsteiner from The Hague). He reported that women who died of eclampsia had agglutinated red cells in their livers.

In 1905, A. Dienst in Germany suggested that these agglutinated cells came from the fetus. He injected methylene blue into the umbilical artery or vein immediately after delivery while the placenta was still attached. Thirty-two of the 160 mothers (22%) passed methylene blue in their urine. Dienst reasoned that the infant's blood, like the methylene blue, had entered the maternal circulation through the placenta. He also demonstrated that the serum of 24 of 118 (20%) of these mothers agglutinated or lysed red cells from their baby.

In 1923, I. McQuarrie studied 180 women with eclampsia, and their children. In 23%, the mothers' plasma agglutinated red cells from their children. In 1923, R. Ottenberg commented that in addition to eclampsia, the jaundice of the newborn "may be due to the same cause, accidental placental transfusion of incompatible blood".

In 1925 and 1926 Ludwig

Hirszfeld compared the consequences of the mother bearing a child with a different ABO type from herself. He measured ABO antibody levels as serological evidence that the placenta was selectively permeable, enabling the fetal blood to enter the mother, and he reasoned that the mother's antibodies might enter the fetus when mother and child were ABO incompatible. He measured the influence on the sex and birth weight of the babies, and understood the likelihood of infant pathology:

> Even when antibodies are passed, they are in the cord blood at lower levels than in the mother . . . our findings make it appear possible that serologically tangible interactions between mother and fetus can bring about some pathological symptoms during pregnancy, but also the future life prospects of the children.

Between 1946 and 1955, many studies demonstrated that normal, elliptocytic, and sickle trait red cells injected into the mother at delivery crossed the placenta. In 1948, Wiener reported a grossly anemic newborn (hemoglobin 7.4 grams/dL), attributing it to a massive placental bleed as there was no evidence of hemolysis or hemorrhage.

In 1954, Bruce Chown reported that in anemic babies there was a lesion in the placenta, which could have been the source of the fetal bleeding. He calculated that in one

Diagnosis of HDN

In developed countries, the maternal plasma is routinely tested at 12 weeks gestation for the presence of antibodies. This testing is done in case the mother has a hemorrhage at delivery requiring a transfusion or the child requires an exchange transfusion in utero or at birth.

If an antibody is detected, its specificity is identified. If it has been described to cause HDN in other women, further blood samples are tested at predetermined intervals for any new antibody specificities and for an increase in antibody strength that would indicate possible HDN.

If a maternal antibody is present, determination of the blood type of the fetus will show if it is at risk for HDN. This used to be predicted by testing blood from the father, or testing fetal red cells obtained from a blood sample collected from the umbilical vein in utero. Such blood sampling is invasive and can harm the fetus. Since the discovery in 1997 that by the second trimester, free fetal DNA is present in the maternal circulation, it provides a non-invasive way to predict the fetal blood group.

When the mother has an antibody to a blood group antigen that the fetal red cells express, the mother should be monitored for signs of fetal distress.

Treatment

TRANSFUSION
From the early 1930s, affected babies were transfused to correct their anemia. These transfusions were of limited value, because Rh-positive blood was often used in ignorance of its unsuitability.

EXCHANGE TRANSFUSION
In the early transfusions blood was first removed to make room for the blood to be transfused, thus conceptually they were not exchange transfusions. In Canada in 1922, there were 122 exchange transfusions for the removal of toxins. In 1923, J.B. Sidbury reported an exchange transfusion using the umbilical vein of a child with hemorrhagic disease of the newborn. In Toronto in 1925, A.P. Hart reported a successful exchange transfusion for the treatment of HDN. In 1946, Harry Wallerstein and Alexander Wiener and Louis Diamond all described an exchange transfusion method.

Diamond bled and then injected blood through a catheter inserted in the umbilical vein; this was adopted widely.

Exchange transfusions were a great improvement over simple transfusion. They removed antibody-bound damaged red cells that survived for a very few days, they removed free maternal antibody in the child's plasma, and removed bilirubin reducing the risk of brain damage, and boosted the hemoglobin level. It became clear that if the unborn baby could be transfused before the devastating effects of red cell destruction occurred, the outcome would be ever better. A second exchange transfusion may be indicated if the bilirubin level is above 20 mg/dL.

INTRAUTERINE TRANSFUSION

In 1956, D.C. Bevis at St Mary's Hospital, London, pioneered amniocentesis. He demonstrated that measurement of bilirubin in the amniotic fluid was a reliable guide for both treatment and prognosis. In 1963, in Auckland, New Zealand, A.W. Liley performed the first intra-uterine blood transfusion on an eight-month-old fetus with a high amniotic bilirubin level. After a second transfusion, the child was delivered by Cesarean section and survived. Today, blood can be given as early as 18 weeks, either intraperitoneally, or intravascularly.

Hydrops is an indication for exchange transfusion, or delivery. Incipient hydrops may be detected by imaging, or it may be inferred from a high amniotic bilirubin level, or a low fetal hemoglobin level that may be determined directly from a blood sample, or indirectly by Doppler ultrasound.

PHOTOTHERAPY

At birth, phototherapy—exposure to blue light at 460 nm—is used to convert unconjugated bilirubin in the skin into a water soluble form that is readily excreted in the bile and urine. The blue light penetrates 0.1 to 1 mm into the skin, where it only reaches a part of the total bilirubin. This followed a ward sister's observation in 1958, that the jaundice in babies briefly exposed to sunlight, faded faster.

Prevention

In 1941, Levine wrote that the most effective way to prevent Rh hemolytic disease would be to manipulate or suppress the immune

case the fetus bled 160–320 mL (5–10 fl. oz), that is about half the total blood volume of an average 7 lb infant.

Marion Lewis used the capillary tube test to demonstrate small differences in the amount of fetal blood in the maternal circulation. In one case, where the mother was type Rh– and her baby was Rh+, Lewis tested the mother's blood with directly agglutinating anti-D. She noted minute agglutinates. To estimate the proportion of D+ fetal red cells present, Lewis made a range of mixtures of D+ and D– red cells and compared the size and number of agglutinates. She estimated the mother's blood had "greater than the 5% but less than the 10% Rh+ in Rh– blood". It was the first direct quantification of fetal red cells in the maternal circulation. These fetal Rh+ red cells stimulated the mother's immune system so that anti-Rh, not detectable at delivery, was found in her plasma a mere 20 days postpartum. This is much earlier than three to four months as is usual after deliberate immunization. Chown inferred that a small number of red cells must have passed from the fetus to the mother throughout her pregnancy, otherwise the rate of maternal anti-Rh production after delivery would not have been so rapid.

Finally, Chown provided evidence that if a fetal bleed at birth is large enough and the mother's plasma contains anti-Rh, it can actually cause a transfusion reaction in the mother.

reaction of the Rh-negative mother. He stated that the chance that it would be achieved in his lifetime was remote. However, in 1943, he provided one important clue when he reported that parents of children with HDN (all with Rh-negative mothers and Rh-positive fathers) were of the same ABO blood group twice as often as expected. Levine explained that:

> There are obviously several factors responsible for fetal death in this group [*erythroblastosis fetalis*], but these preliminary studies strongly suggest that at least one of them will be found to be isoimmunization of the mother by the incompatible A or B of the fetus.

In 1950, Race and Sanger cited five subsequent studies, all with a similar conclusion. They wrote that:

> If Rh sensitization is due to foetal red cells entering the maternal circulation, it seems possible that if they carry, for example the A antigen, and the maternal serum carries anti-A, then these invading cells may be eliminated before they have time to act as an Rh antigen.

Levine's finding regarding the protective effect of ABO incompatibility provoked studies of 429 families by H.R. Nevanlinna, and T. Vainio in Finland (1956), 91 families by C.A. Clarke, R. Finn, and R.B. McConnell in England (1958), and several other studies. They all confirmed Levine's finding.

MODIFICATION OF IMMUNE RESPONSE

At the meeting of the American Association of Blood Banks in San Francisco in August 1960, K. Stern, H. Goodman, and M. Berger presented results of ingenious experiments, these being published in 1961. They had injected Rh-negative men with Rh-positive blood to demonstrate that antibody production was lower in those whose ABO group did not match the injected blood. However, in those injected with matching ABO (compatible ABO but incompatible Rh), when the Rh-positive red cells were first coated in vitro with Rh antibodies, none provoked Rh antibodies, whereas uncoated Rh-positive red cells stimulated Rh antibody production in half of the subjects. The concept of suppressing Rh antibody production with Rh antibody, was the basis of their grant application approved by NIH in 1959.

Two teams

By 1960, a transatlantic competition to prevent Rh HDN started between three New Yorkers and a group in Liverpool, England, headed by Cyril Clarke, who attributed the success of their "useless research" to:

> team spirit engendered from collective amateurism . . . no members of the team were pediatricians or obstetricians, and we played no part in the management of patients with rhesus disease . . .

Clarke was professor of medicine at Liverpool, and was influenced by Philip Sheppard, an Oxford geneticist who joined his team in 1956. In 1952, Sheppard had advertised in the *Amateur Entomologist's Bulletin* for Swallowtail butterfly pupae and Clarke, who was also an amateur lepidopterist, replied that he could hand mate them. Having trained at Oxford with E.B. Ford, Sheppard believed that blood groups were maintained by selection, which led to work with Clarke on the association of blood groups and disease, and then to the study of HDN. They thought, falsely, that Rh in man, and mimicry in the swallowtails, were both controlled by supergenes that were modified by ABO and sex, respectively.

When Clarke's senior house officer, Ronald Finn, asked for suggestions for a research project, Clarke proposed that he use the local Liverpool population to confirm the protective effect of ABO on HDN. When interviewed, Finn explained:

> I was SHO [Senior House Officer] during the day, I worked doing family studies every evening, [1956–1958] finding the ABO status of all the Rh incompatible women. Then just by luck, Kleihauer published his paper [15 June 1957] and I then switched my evening work to look at transplacental leakage. It was soon obvious that when there were [fetal] cells women became sensitized, where there were no fetal cells they were not sensitized. I could predict which ones would become sensitized, finding evidence of fetal bleeds in about one third of the ABO compatible matings and in none of the incompatible matings.

Kleihauer's method eluted adult but not fetal hemoglobin from

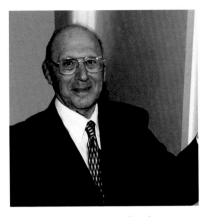

Fig. 6.1 Ronald Finn after he received the Lasker Award shared with Cyril Clarke, Vince Freda, John Gorman and Bill Pollack in 1980; in 1946 the award was given to Karl Landsteiner, Alexander Wiener and Philip Levine

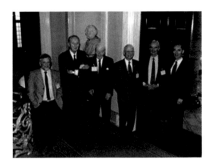

Fig. 6.2 Left to right: Nevin Hughes-Jones, Patrick Mollison Cyril Clarke, and colleagues

red cells, so that maternal red cells appear as retractile empty ghosts, whereas fetal red cells remain intact. In 1959, using a small modification of the Kleihauer method, Zipursky demonstrated that blood from 21% of 42 mothers after delivery had at least one fetal red cell per low power field, while one mother had 16 fetal red cells per low power field. Finn switched to the Zipursky method. He found that only one in twenty pregnancies of an Rh-negative woman with an Rh-positive husband produced a child with HDN, which suggested that there was a natural protective mechanism in the other 19. In concordance with others, Finn confirmed fetal cells in the maternal blood in one third of ABO compatible couples but in none in the ABO incompatible couples 72 hours postpartum, confirming that fetal red cells were removed from the maternal circulation by anti-A or anti-B. He reported this to the local medical society on February 18, 1960:

> It might be possible to destroy any fetal red cells found in the maternal circulation following delivery by means of a suitable antibody.

2. In 2003, Sir David Weatherall asked Finn about the dream story: "Do you think there is any possibility that that was true?" Finn replied that he had not given it a thought until a few days ago, but having now done so, he suggested that Clarke never lied. However, the idea went from Finn to Clarke to Féo who forgot about it until it returned to her in a dream, who then told Clarke who had forgotton that it had originated from Finn. Perhaps Finn had in mind George Mikes' observation that "in England people almost never lie, but they are almost never quite honest with you either". Finn's explanation was a good try, but eureka moments are not forgotten. When Darrow had her flash of insight she immediately wrote a 37 page article, and when Winbaum (p. 55), had his, he wrote about it to everyone.

This quote appeared in the Medical Societies section of *The Lancet* on March 5, 1960. The article was a 150–word summary of Finn's 10–minute presentation two weeks earlier at the medical school. Clarke later explained: "All we wanted was priority over the workers in the United States who were on our tails." Thereby confirming that he knew of John Gorman's ideas or Kurt Stern's experiments before they had been published weakening Clarke's claim that the idea was his. Some 40 years later, Finn could not recall whether at the end of his talk, he had stated that anti-Rh was the suitable antibody that he had in mind, but even if he did not say so, he had the idea and it was his. Clarke claimed that Finn got the idea from him, that he was given the idea from his wife Féo, and she received it in a dream.[2]

The first mention in print that anti-D was the suitable antibody was May 27, 1961 in the *British Medical Journal*. Finn, Clarke and team reported the effect of 10 mL anti-D serum injected intravenously into three male volunteers half an hour after an injection of 5 mL of tagged Rh-positive blood. Two days later about half of the injected cells could not be found, whereas there was no loss in the three unprotected controls. They stated that for the prevention of maternal sensitization, "the injection of anti-D would be the first thing to try." If indeed they had conceived in

February 1960 that anti-D was the first thing to try, it is not clear why they did not do so, sitting on their hands for more than a year. They then conducted a two–week experiment on six people. In this 1961 report they referred to the prior publication of their idea in an article in *Nature* (Finn, et al. 1960), which, to our surprise, we have been unable to find.

It could be that the dismissive attitude of colleagues combined with a natural hesitancy in advancing a counter-intuitive concept, accounts for the year's delay in publication. While no one manages to be as objective about their own ideas as they are of their neighbor's, Finn was a straightforward, unassuming person. Moreover, there is some verification of their having had the idea in 1960; an extant copy of a typescript of a talk that Finn gave to the Genetical Society in July 1960 ends:

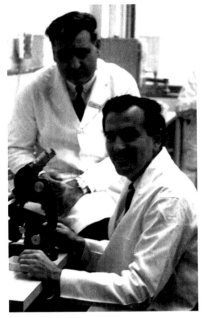

> May I conclude on a highly speculative note: if immunization does in fact occur at delivery, and is due to the presence of Rhesus positive Foetal cells in the maternal circulation, then it may be possible to destroy them by means of a powerful anti-D, and hence artificially prevent immunization, thus mimicing [*sic*] the natural protection afforded by A. B. O. [*sic*] incompatibility.

Fig. 6.3 Vince Freda and John Gorman

The US competition

The American team comprised John Gorman, Vince Freda, and William Pollack. Gorman was an Australian blood bank specialist who trained at Columbia Presbyterian Medical Center in New York; Freda was an obstetrician, an ex-flight surgeon who had trained at New York University Medical School; and Pollack was an English immunologist, with a PhD from Rutgers, who was working at Ortho under Philip Levine. The three met by chance in 1959 or 1960 in New York, and decided to prevent HDN by suppressing the maternal production of antibodies following the method of Theodore Smith[3] that John Gorman had just read in Florey's *General Pathology,* published by Saunders in 1958. Gorman recalls:

> The Saunders salesman came in and we were teaching pathology to the medical students in the lab and so forth, and he gave me a free copy of the book, and he figured that

3. Theodore Smith, 1859-1934, from Albany, NY, found the tick-borne protozoan responsible for Texas fever in 1889—it was the first time an arthropod was found to transmit an infectious disease. He anticipated mosquitoes as vectors of malaria in 1899, discovered anaphylaxis in 1903 and the suppression of active immunity in 1909. Paul Ehrlich in 1900 raised antibodies in rabbits injected with ox blood but when the ox blood was injected together with specific antiserum, antibody production was suppressed.

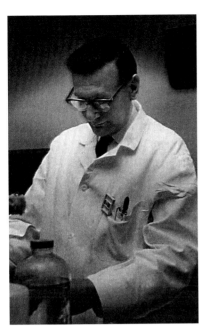

Fig. 6.4 William Pollack

I would recommend it to the students, it was an important book . . . it goes into this passive antibody preventing the active antibody. The book had a chapter by Glenny and Sudmus that summarized Smith's observation that mixtures of diphtheria toxin and antitoxin would suppress immunization in guinea-pigs. Smith wrote: "An excess of anti-toxin reduces the possibility of producing an active immunity and may extinguish it altogether. . . I had met Vince Freda, an obstetrician, at Columbia, Freda was a protégé of Alexander Wiener. Freda had spent his residency at NYU with Wiener. He [Freda] was wonderful, he made it happen, without him, there was no way it would have happened.

Gorman suggested that Smith's modification of antibody response might be applied to HDN, Freda was receptive, for he had been thinking along similar lines, as one can infer from his article:

Nature provides a very good example of this with pregnancy where the baby inherits passively derived immunity from the mother against polio, typhoid, and tetanus. It is extremely difficult to immunize the baby against these, because of the passive immunity derived from the mother. It is not because the baby is unable or incapable of forming antibody. Some years ago, Dr Wolf and I did a small experiment using flocculus antigens on newborns in various stages of pregnancies 7 months to term and found that the babies responded very well with antibody production. Around 1960, it occurred to Dr John Gorman, Dr William Pollack of the Ortho Research Foundation and myself that perhaps we might use this concept and attempt to prevent active immunization of the Rh-negative mother by passive administration of antibody in the third stage of labor.

The New Yorkers' concept of suppressing the immune response by passive administration of anti-D to the mother first appeared in print as a grant application in May 1961, although it had been the basis of their grant proposals submitted to NIH in 1960 and also a paper submitted to Science in 1960. Both were rejected.

The third member of the team, Bill Pollack, began making anti-Rh immunoglobulin (IgG) and by 1961 it was ready for use; it was safe, it was highly concentrated, and the antiglobulin titer was over 200,000. Ignoring the scorn of their colleagues, the New

Yorkers decided to give Rh IgG to suppress immunization. First they tested their hypothesis on volunteer prisoners at a maximum security prison in the erstwhile village of Sing Sing, Ossining, New York.

They injected men with Rh IgG and Rh-positive red cells, and for two years studied their immune response. Initially nine Rh-negative volunteers were injected intravenously with 2 mL of Rh-positive red cells every month. Four of the nine were given 5 mL Rh IgG intramuscularly 24 hours before the red cells, each dose containing 7,500 µg anti-Rh. This was repeated monthly for one year. Subsequently, an additional 27 volunteers were added; all were given two injections of 10 mL of Rh-positive red cells at six-month intervals, and 72 hours later, 14 of them were given Rh IgG intramuscularly. Of the 18 who had been given Rh IgG, none were sensitized; of the 18 unprotected controls, 12 were sensitized. There were no cases of hepatitis and no allergic reactions. After a further year of tests to determine whether antibody production had occurred, not one had been sensitized, there was no untoward reaction and no morbidity. They began a clinical trial in April 1964.

The decision to test the efficacy of anti-D three days after the injection of Rh-positive red cells was made by the warden of Sing Sing because he feared that a return visit two days in a row, ran a risk of attempted prison escapes. The warden's alteration of their anti-D injection protocol from immediate to 72 hours delay was lucky and logistically extremely helpful, because it established that Rh IgG would give effective protection up to 72 hours after antigenic exposure.

When Rh IgG suppressed immunization in the Sing Sing inmates, John Gorman decided to prevent sensitization in his nine-month pregnant sister-in-law Kath. She was Rh-negative, her husband, John's brother, was Rh-positive, and they were both living in London. Bill Pollack supplied Rh IgG to John who took it to the recently renamed JFK airport. His brother and sister-in-law collected it at Heathrow airport. One day later, on January 31st, 1964, Kath Gorman became the first woman in the world to have received Ortho's purified Rh IgG; it prevented sensitization despite a 5 mL transplacental bleed. John Gorman added: "She had 5 more Rh-positive babies, covered with Rh immune globulin, and has remained unsensitized." Clarke immediately wrote a terminologically inexact letter to the Lancet, implying that Kath Gorman was part of the Liverpool project, that the initiative came from Australia and he forgot to mention the New Yorkers:

She is a member of a medical family and her father-in-law in Australia, being familiar with the progress made in the experimental studies, and knowing that she might be at risk, had some American anti-D gamma globulin flown over for her.

On April 13, 1963, the Liverpudlians published a study on male volunteers similar to the one at Sing Sing except that the anti-Rh was raw serum. To their surprise, the experiments conducted showed that this approach did not suppress immunization, indeed it enhanced it. However, when they learned that the New York team was achieving success with concentrated IgG anti-D, they asked if they could have some, which Bill Pollack supplied.

In 1965, Clarke's team reported results of a study of ten Rh-negative post-menopausal women given Rh IgG prepared from pooled sera of 11 hyperimmunized male volunteers half an hour after being injected with tagged Rh-positive blood drawn from the umbilical vein of three babies. The result on the women was the same as the men. They also reported the preliminary results of a maternal study started in May 1964 in which they used Rh IgG on alternate high risk mothers, that is, those who were Rh incompatible, ABO compatible and with a fetal-cell score of five or greater. They found that:

> After five months three out of eight controls have produced immune antibodies . . . In contrast none of the six treated women has yet produced any evidence of immune anti-D formation.

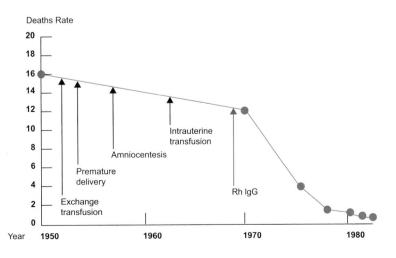

Fig. 6.5 Perinatal deaths due to HDN per 10,000 from 1950 showing the benefits of progressive improvements in treatment plus prevention

Major trials were also started in St. Louis, Missouri in 1962, in New York City, NY in 1964, in Manitoba, Canada at the beginning of 1965, in Scotland, Freiburg, Germany and in several other countries. At a meeting in a hotel in 1965 in New York, the results were announced, creating excitement rather like an election convention: New York, 34 treated, no sensitizations; Liverpool, 27 treated, no sensitizations; California, 22 treated, no sensitizations; Winnipeg, 4 treated, no sensitizations. In all studies, about a quarter of the controls were sensitized. One startling result came from Zipursky who reported that it was safe and effective to give Rh IgG during pregnancy. By 1966, the results confirmed that IgG anti-D prevented immunization. On March 28, 1967 Freda reported:

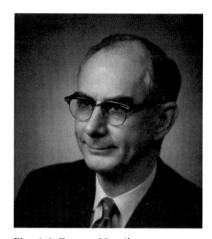

Fig. 6.6 Eugene Hamilton

> 444 mothers who have received RhoGAM [Ortho's Rh IgG] who have been followed for six months up to three years, none are actively immunized to Rh. We have 469 untreated mothers, 58 are actively immunized to Rh. Of the 444 mothers, 37 have gone on to have another Rh-positive infant. None of the mothers are sensitized; no affected baby. Of 469 [controls], 34 have had another Rh-positive infant. 10 mothers are actively immunized to Rh. 10 babies were affected with Rh hemolytic disease of the newborn.

Using Nevin Hughes-Jones invaluable method of estimating anti-D, Mollison (1969) established the recommended dose to inhibit the development of active immunity. In 1973, J.C. Woodrow, a member of Clarke's team, summarized the data from all the major studies with the number of women in parentheses: Finland (12,720), USA (3,389), Germany (3,091), Canada (2,247), Sweden (2,214), Holland (1,563), and England (526). The results consistently demonstrated that sensitization could be prevented and thus also, the disease.

Prenatal HDN prevention

Mollison's strategy is given in his book:

1. Ensure that no Rh-negative woman is missed because she is classified as Rh-positive. Test for Rh antigen at least once during pregnancy and at delivery to assess the size of the placental bleed.

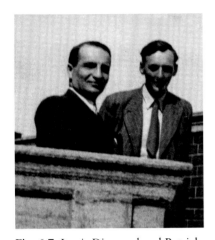

Fig. 6.7 Louis Diamond and Patrick Mollison

2. All Rh-negative women with Rh-positive infants should be given Rh IgG after delivery, abortions, amniocentesis, versions, abdominal trauma, Cesarean section, ectopic pregnancies, forceps delivery, and placental biopsy.

3. Following delivery, measure the number of fetal red cells in the mother's blood to determine if the bleed was large enough to warrant more Rh IgG. This overcomes failure due to a fetal bleed that is larger than the antibody can protect against. The second source of failure is due to fetal bleeds during pregnancy, before Rh IgG has been given. This could be overcome by giving Rh IgG during pregnancy.

4. It is curious that the plasma used by Hamilton in USA apparently worked in preventing active anti-D immunization while plasma used by the UK group did not. It is not surprising that the material used by the New York and Winnipeg groups worked, as it was concentrated IgG. It is therefore tempting to speculate that the plasma used by Hamilton worked because it was from women with the most severe disease—stillborn hydropic babies—who had high levels of IgG. His success with raw plasma was also attributable to his ignorance of the 72 hour rule. and was fortified by the willingness of women with an HDN baby to donate plasma to help prevent the devastating disease. As anti-D production in women was prevented by injections of anti-D, HDN became a rare condition and the source of anti-D dwindled. Today, anti-D with sufficient titer is obtained from Rh-negative males who volunteer to be immunized with D-positive red cells (matched for all other blood group antigens).

Eugene Hamilton (1910 –2005)

There is no country in the world, outside the USA, that exhibits such independence of spirit and self reliance to produce the like of Dr Eugene Hamilton, the St. Louis obstetrician (Fig 6.6) who was a member of Gorman's audience in 1967 when Gorman was lecturing to explain the success in preventing HDN. Hamilton stood up to explain that he already knew of the efficiency of passive immunity for preventing HDN as he had conducted his own clinical trial of anti-Rh. It was the world's first and at that time about ten times larger than the English trial. On reading the articles by Finn et al. (1961) and Stern et al. (1961) and editorials on them, he had decided to prepare his own Rh antibody[4] rather than deprive his patients for years while awaiting the development of commercial pooled plasma with its attendant risks. He identified ten well motivated Rh-negative mothers who had delivered stillborn babies with hydrops. They had been followed for several years during which time they had been free of hepatitis and other communicable diseases. He then withdrew about 450 mL blood from each, separated the plasma, and stored it in 10 mL sterile aliquots that were kept frozen until needed. Over a ten year period, beginning April 1, 1962, he injected 3–10 mL high titered anti-D plasma (almost always intramuscularly) into Rh-negative mothers as soon as possible, but within 72 hours of delivery. Over ten years he had injected 1,400 women without any adverse effects. Of these, 240 returned for 336 subsequent Rh-positive babies. Of these, three developed HDN, two were so mild that they required no treatment, and one developed hydrops and died. Of his 88 untreated control mothers who delivered Rh positive babies, sixteen were sensitized.

Genetic counseling

Genetic counseling which offers a way to sidestep an enormous amount of human misery, is not being utilized widely by society . . . The counselor should not shirk his responsibility in explaining the risks and the management procedures, but the prospective parents must be allowed to make the final decision.

—John Gorman, 1975

The Wellcome Witness Seminar in 2003 entitled "The Rhesus Factor and Disease Prevention" was intended to provide historians with new insights and reveal from the horse's mouth how the discoveries came about. All clinicians and researchers who had played a part in HDN were invited to take part in this oral history—all that is, except the Americans: Gorman, Pollack and Hamilton were not invited, and no-one raised Darrow's ideas on eugenics or on the etiology.

After Ruth Darrow's first affected son died, she had considered artificial insemination by which it is possible to reduce the risk of HDN to zero, and in a letter to the *Journal of the American Medical Association*, in 1945, Darrow wrote:

Potter recently reported the production of an unaffected child by the artificial insemination of an Rh-negative woman with semen from an Rh-negative man.

When Sir David Weatherall, who chaired the Wellcome Seminar, moved the topic of the discussion to eugenics, he asked Patrick Mollison[5] for his opinion at that time:

Weatherall: Were there any thoughts about prevention for the future?
Mollison: I think the idea of artificial insemination from Rh-negative men was certainly discussed. It was quite a lively topic at one time.
Weatherall: That was your idea, was it?
Mollison: No, no.

5. We interviewed Professor Mollison in his home shortly before his 90th birthday. We found a modest, upright, companionable gentleman whose unsurpassed book *Blood Transfusion in Clinical Medicine* has biblical status in transfusion medicine. In addition, he developed acid-dextrose-citrate anticoagulant (with J.F. Loutit, and I.M. Young), established criteria for measuring the severity of HDN, quantified IgG anti-D (with Nevin Hughes-Jones), evaluated the results of the clinical trials, and determined the optimal dose to prevent immunization. He found the first anti-K in a mother whose baby had HDN without anti-D. He cared for Mr Duffy, a multi-transfused hemophiliac who became jaundiced after a transfusion of Rh-negative blood. When plasma from Mr Duffy was tested with random blood donors, the prevalence was different from known antigens. The antibody was named anti-Fy[a].

In 1947, Mollison was the first person in the UK to do an exchange transfusion using plastic catheters. Louis Diamond had lectured in London and the two men struck up a friendship. Diamond left his equipment, which was a vast improvement over what Mollison had been using. Aside from the nine editions of his book, the achievement for which he was most proud was measuring the effect of different antibodies on the survival of small amounts of Cr51-labelled red cells. Complement binding antibodies have a different effect on clearance. IgG antibodies like anti-D were cleared in the spleen.

Mollison had been a medical student at St. Thomas Hospital, London. He said that during the war, under qualified, he was sent to India. He served in Bengal, in West Africa, and then in Burma before he was de-mobbed in 1946, with the rank of Colonel. He set up the British Blood Transfusion Service in one of the three Medical Research Council blood depots, he moved to the Post Graduate Medical Unit where Marie Cutbush (later Crookston) joined him as a valued assistant.

Results of immunization

Use of Rh IgG to prevent active immunity to the D antigen has dramatically reduced mortality and morbidity. Today HDN is rare, but it can be caused by almost any IgG antibody. Table 6.1 shows the percentage decrease of fetal deaths in Manitoba, Canada following each management strategy.

Table 6.1 Effect of clinical management on HDN

Date	Clinical Management	Death Rate
Before 1942	None	50%
1942–1952	Exchange transfusion	25%
1954–1961	Selective induction	16%
1963–1964	Intrauterine fetal transfusion	8%
1969–1975	IgG injection at delivery	3%
1975–1983	IgG injection at 28 weeks	0.5%

The following seem to us the most significant contributions in the conquest of HDN:

1905 **Dienst** discovered that the placenta can leak blood.

1923 **Ottenberg** proposed that the placenta leaked blood in HDN, provoking maternal antibodies.

1931 **Ferguson** brought together all the clinical manifestations of HDN into one disease.

1938 **Darrow** recognized all the essential elements of the disease. She postulated a fetal antigen that immunized the mother. The antibodies then destroyed the child's red cells.

1939 **Levine** discovered a blood group that he soon thought was the Rh blood group.

1940 **Landsteiner and Wiener** discovered a new blood group by injecting the blood of Rhesus monkeys into rabbits. They called it Rh.

1940 **Wiener and Peters** reported four intragroup transfusion reactions attributable to the donor's Rh incompatibility. From a review of published cases, they noted that transfusion reactions that occurred at the first transfusion only occurred in women, such as Mrs Seno, and they postulated that a prior blood donor or the fetus had provided the Rh antigen.

1943   **Levine** discovered that ABO incompatibility varied inversely with HDN.

1954   **Lewis and Chown** demonstrated that fetal red cells passed into the maternal circulation.

1957   **Winbaum** conceived the counter-intuitive idea of injecting the mother with anti-Rh at delivery, the very same antibody that she had produced, that had destroyed the child's red cells.

1959   **Zipursky** demonstrated that placental bleeding occurs in at least 21% of deliveries.

1960   **Stern, Goodman, and Berger** demonstrated that Rh positive red cells coated with Rh IgG were not antigenic. **Finn, Freda and Gorman** conceived passive immunization of the mother with Rh IgG to prevent sensitization.

1961   **Pollack** processed Rh IgG.

1962   **Hamilton** started the first clinical trial.

1965   **Zipursky** demonstrated that antenatal Rh IgG surppressed sensitization and was harmless to the fetus.

The concept of using anti-Rh was particularly praise-worthy because it went against current thinking. It was initially opposed by Chown, Allen, Levine, Wiener, Mollison and all the experts. Finn, Clarke, McConnell, Woodrow, Gorman, Freda, and Pollack showed great courage to conceive that it was feasible, and push it through despite opposition. Gorman's use of Rh IgG on his sister-in-law in 1964 was indeed courageous. Even after the effectiveness of Bill Pollack's Rh IgG was proven on volunteers, experts feared to use it during pregnancy; a fear heightened by the discovery in 1961 that thalidomide given during pregnancy had deformed 8,000 babies.

It is hard to know whether the letters that Edward Winbaum wrote to many experts in 1957 were dismissed as worthless nonsense or whether some experts like Sydney Gellis, or Fred Allen (see below), had thought it an interesting but a perverse point of view; that was, on reflection, true, so that it permeated the scientific consciousness, and emerged in 1960 as Féo's dream. In 1968, the editor of *Pediatrics* published the following correspondence entitled 'Immunization of Rh-negative Mother with Rh Antisera'.

To the Editor:

After reading Dr. Diamond's article on the history and advances made against erythroblastosis [Louis K. Diamond. Protection Against Rh Sensitization And Prevention Of Erythroblastosis Fetalis, *Pediatrics* 1968;41:1–4], I am encouraged to submit (with his approval) a copy of a letter dated August 23, 1957, received from Dr. S. Gellis in reply to an idea which came to me about 11 years ago. The general pediatrician might consider it an interesting footnote to the "erythroblastosis story" and perhaps be more persevering in his own original thoughts. I might add that Dr. Gellis's reply was the only encouraging response verbal or written, from many opinions received.

Edward S. Winbaum M.D.
1027 Ottawa Street, Windsor
Ontario, Canada

Editor's note: Doctor Gellis's reply, somewhat worn in the creases by now, was as follows:

To the best of my knowledge no one has ever tried to passively immunize an Rh-negative mother with Rh antisera given immediately after birth. It would probably work and it is a good suggestion. To prove its efficacy would be a bit of work. I discussed your letter with Dr. Fred Allen of the Boston Blood Grouping Lab., who agreed with me that no one has tried to do this. He and I both will be very glad to offer advice or help should you wish to try it out. I asked Dr. Allen why he didn't try it himself and he answered that he has so many projects going that he has no time at present. He admitted that several of these are not as worthwhile as the one you have suggested.

Sydney S. Gellis, MD.

Chapter 7   **More Antigens Revealed**

> What's in a name? That which we call a rose, by any
> other word would smell as sweet.
>
> —William Shakespeare

Between 1940 and 1945, while World War II was raging, several more antibodies and antigens were identified and it was during this time that the way in which blood group antigens were named changed.

Once it was recognized that an antibody to a blood group antigen was the cause of HDN, plasma samples from women who had delivered babies with HDN were tested against a set of red cells from individuals known to be type Rh+ or Rh−. While plasma from some women gave an identical pattern of reactions with the set of typed red cells, plasma from other women gave different, but clearly related, patterns (Table 7.1). Thus, it became obvious that other antibody specificities existed.

Table 7.1 Results of testing a plasma against Rh+ and Rh− red cells

D Type	Pattern with anti-D	New Pattern
+	+	+
+	+	+
+	+	−
+	+	−
−	−	+
−	−	−
−	−	−
−	−	−

The original Rh antigen was renamed as Rh_0 by Wiener in the USA, and as D by Race in the UK. Because the name Rh was so entrenched, it has persisted to this day: blood is labeled as Rh+ or Rh– and not D+ or D– as would be expected since the red cells are tested with anti-D.

Rh expands

In 1941, using the direct agglutination test (see Fig. 5.1), an antibody that gave a novel pattern of positive (agglutinated) and negative (non-agglutinated) reactions was found in the plasma of a woman whose baby had HDN. Most red cells that were agglutinated were D+ and only rare examples were D–, thus the new antibody was clearly detecting an antigen related to D. This antibody agglutinated 70% of red cell samples from random donors (anti-D agglutinated 85%) and was originally called anti-70%. Landsteiner and Wiener named this antibody: anti-rh′ and the antigen: rh′.

Landsteiner and Wiener used an upper case "R" and a subscript "0", to distinguish anti-Rh_0 from the other Rh antibodies and to indicate its special clinical importance. They assigned lower case letters and superscripts for the other Rh antigens: rh′, rh″, and hr′. Why they used prime and double-prime is not documented. The reversing of rh to hr was used for antithetical antigens (i.e. encoded by alternative alleles); similarly rh′ and hr′ are antithetical.

Concurrently, virtually parallel studies were being performed in England by Rob Race. He named the original "anti-Rh" as anti-D, and anti-70% (anti-rh′) as anti-C. The other two "Rh" antibodies were named anti-E (anti-rh″) and anti-c (anti-hr′). These symbols were chosen to avoid confusion with any symbols so far used (A, B, O, M, N, P).

To understand the relationship of these antigens, in 1943/44, Race consulted the geneticist, R.A. Fisher, Chair of the Department of Genetics, Cambridge. He noted that the antigens, C and c, were clearly antithetical (see Table 7.2). The reactions of anti-D and anti-E were not antithetical, and were clearly different from the reactions of anti-C and anti-c. Fisher postulated that D and E also had antithetical antigens, which would be capable, in favorable circumstances, of stimulating their own antibodies, anti-d and anti-e. Anti-e was indeed later found but anti-d was not.

The priority, terminology, and genetics of Rh were disputed. As the Wiener Rh terminology was complex and cumbersome, the Fisher/Race terminology quickly became more popular and was eventually accepted universally. Wiener believed there was one gene

Table 7.2 Results of testing a plasma against red cells typed for the known Rh antigens (four D+ and four D−)

Antigen type				Patterns of agglutination obtained with plasma containing			
D	C	c	E	Anti-D	Anti-C	Anti-c	Anti-E
+	+	−	−	+	+	−	−
+	+	−	−	+	+	−	−
+	−	+	+	+	−	+	+
+	−	+	+	+	−	+	+
−	+	+	−	−	+	+	−
−	−	+	+	−	−	+	+
−	−	+	−	−	−	+	−
−	−	+	−	−	−	+	−

that encoded antigens in the Rh family, while Fisher/Race believed there were three closely linked genes. Today, we know that neither was correct and that there are in fact two closely linked genes that encode the Rh antigens. One gene, *RHD*, encodes the RhD protein, on which are expressed many parts of the D antigen. An absence of *RHD* is an amorph, that is, a deleted gene or one with no phenotypic effect: no protein is produced and the red cells type as D−. For this reason, there cannot be an altered gene encoding an antithetical antigen, which explains why a d antigen has not been, and will not be, found. The second gene, *RHCE*, encodes the RhCE protein that expresses C or c and E or e. Rh is now known to comprise more than 50 antigens, although only four (D, C, E, and c) were initially revealed using the direct agglutination test.

Lutteran or Lutheran?

In 1946, another antibody, anti-Luᵃ, was found by the direct agglutination test in the plasma of a patient with systemic lupus erythematosus who had been transfused nine times for persistent anemia. One of the blood donors, Mr Lutteran, stimulated production of an antibody that was named anti-Lutheran. It had been hard to read the handwriting on the tube of blood that was sent to

Race's laboratory for investigation and the name "Lutteran" was misread as "Lutheran". The name stuck. The superscript "a" was used even though the antithetical antigen had not been discovered. Anti-Lu^a/Lu^a was the first antibody/antigen combination to be given a name that was derived from the name of the donor whose red cells expressed the antigen. This started a trend. Subsequently, several antibody/antigen pairs were named either after the donor whose red cells expressed the antigen or after the first patient in whose plasma the antibody was found. This has led to a colorful array of names. While a name is merely a label, a good name improves communication, and unambiguous communication is essential in transfusion medicine (See Chapter 10).

Lewis antigen

Also in 1946, Arthur Mourant found Le^a. The name Le^a, was derived from Lewis, the last name of one of the two original producers of anti-Le^a. Lewis antigens (Le^a and Le^b) are carbohydrates attached to lipids that are adsorbed onto the red cell membrane from plasma. They are not integral to the red cell membrane. This phenomenon was shown in an elegantly simple experiment. The husband and wife team of Peter and Joan Sneath incubated red cells lacking Le^b antigen [type Le(a+b−)] in plasma from an Le(b+) person. The red cells lost their Le^a antigen and gained the Le^b antigen, and thus typed Le(a−b+). This marvel is useful in transfusion; patients with anti-Le^b in their plasma have been safely transfused with Le(b+) blood because the transfused red cells acquire the Lewis type of the recipient.

Evidence for inadequacy of test method

By the mid 1940s, it was clear that antibodies to other blood group antigens must exist. Why? Because there were many cases of HDN and many transfusion reactions that could not be attributed to any known blood group that was detectable by the direct agglutination test. A different detection method was needed.

Chapter 8

The Coombs Revolution

> That's one small step for [a] man, one giant leap for mankind.
>
> — Neil Armstrong

Robin Coombs, a Londoner who in 1945 conceived a revolutionary technique, thought his contribution was merely a small step, yet everyone in the field would consider it one giant leap for mankind. Until 1945, red cells had always been typed for blood group antigens by the direct agglutination test.

The direct agglutination test is a single stage procedure (Figs. 5.1 and 8.4). We now know that antigens that are detected by this test (ABO, M, N, and P1) are abundant on red cell membranes. The indirect (Coombs) agglutination test is a two stage procedure. The test, like the direct test, can be used in different ways:

(a) Red cells of known type can be mixed with unknown plasma to determine which antibodies are present in the plasma,

(b) Red cells of unknown type can be mixed with plasma containing a known antibody, to determine the type of the red cells,

(c) Without knowing the identity of either the antigen or the antibody (as in the crossmatch), the absence or presence of agglutination is a good indicator that they do or do not match. In the crossmatch, a patient's plasma is tested against donor red cells to detect incompatibility between donor blood and a recipient, thereby showing which donor blood should not be transfused—to prevent a transfusion reaction.

By 1940, however, it had became apparent that the direct test did not detect all antibodies. Soon after the discovery of anti-Rh, investigators realized that other antibodies must exist that could not be explained on the basis of known blood groups. The presence of antibodies was inferred because the patient was a better litmus test than the direct agglutination test.

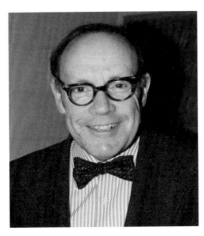

Fig. 8.1 Professor Robert Royston Amos (Robin) Coombs FRS

In an attempt to detect these inferred antibodies, investigators tried numerous variations on the basic direct agglutination test. They tried different support environments (e.g. tiles, slides, tubes), different temperatures (4°C, 24°C, 37°C), and different ratios of plasma to red cells (using an increased volume of plasma to red cells, and different concentrations of red cells). These attempts had some success but failed to achieve a satisfactory degree of sensitivity. Bruce Chown and Marion Lewis at the Rh Laboratory in Winnipeg achieved pretty good results by mixing red cells, plasma, and bovine albumin in a capillary tube. They were able to detect antibody/antigen reactions not detected by direct agglutination; however, even this technique did not detect all the antibodies that were thought to occur. Simply mixing plasma and red cells to detect an antibody to a blood group antigen was not enough—something was missing.

Incomplete or blocking antibodies, not detectable by direct tests

By 1941, A.S. Wiener had accumulated several plasma samples containing "non-detectable" antibodies. He developed an ingenious method of demonstrating their presence. He first mixed plasma containing the no-longer-reactive anti-Rh (as in, for example Mrs Seno) with Rh+ red cells. As expected, nothing visible happened. He then added plasma containing a direct agglutinating anti-Rh, which now failed to agglutinate the red cells. He, rightly, inferred the Rh+ sites on the red cells were blocked by the non-detectable anti-Rh bound to the Rh antigens; he called them "blocking" antibodies. Wiener also referred to the blocking antibodies as "Rh glutinin", derived from "half an agglutinin". Although the name did not catch on, it reflects his concept that these antibodies might be too small to attach to two different red cells to cause agglutination but quite capable of attaching to a single red cell and blocking the antigen site. Using his "blocking test", Wiener was able to demonstrate the presence of anti-Rh in plasma from mothers of babies with HDN. However, the test was difficult to perform.

In England, Rob Race had made similar observations and called these antibodies "incomplete", comparing them to the "complete" (or direct) agglutinating type. It soon became clear that the non-agglutinating anti-Rh antibodies were present in

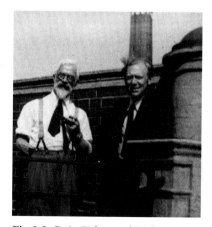

Fig 8.2 R.A. Fisher and Robert Race on the Cambridge Pathology Department roof where the Blood Group Research unit was housed during WW II.

plasma from some women whose babies had HDN and from patients with unexplained transfusion reactions. These non-agglutinating anti-Rh were more significant clinically than the direct or complete agglutinating type. Due to blocking, some babies with HDN had red cells that typed (falsely) Rh-negative. However, by using the blocking test, it was shown that these babies were indeed Rh-positive. Blocking or incomplete anti-Rh antibodies bound to the babies' red cells prevented the reagent anti-Rh from agglutinating them.

Antibodies are immunoglobulins

At the University of Uppsala, Sweden, Theodor Svedberg won the Nobel Prize in Chemistry in 1926 in part for inventing the ultracentrifuge to measure the size of molecules. He said: "Once one has become convinced of the existence of atoms and molecules, the question as to their real size is naturally a question of the very greatest interest." In 1937, he separated proteins into three groups by size and suggested that it indicated that proteins had a modular structure. In 1930, his assistant Arne Tiselius developed electrophoresis (a process to separate proteins dissolved in a gel medium by passing an electrical current though it); it led to a Nobel Prize in 1948, also in Chemistry. Arne Tiselius and Elvin Kabat had shown that most of the "non-detectable" antibodies were in the 7S portion and were globulins. The ultracentrifuge was capable of separating the globulins into two groups, one with a sedimentation rate of 7S, and another 19S (S is a Svedberg unit of time, 10^{-13} seconds). Bigger particles tend to sediment faster and have higher Svedberg units. Two decades later, because antibodies are globulins produced by the immune system, they were renamed immunoglobulins, abbreviated to Ig. The 7S fraction became IgG (G from gamma) and the 19S fraction became IgM (M from macroglobulin). The various names for these two classes of antibodies are given in Fig. 8.3.

The Coombs concept

In 1945 Robin Coombs, a 24-year-old PhD student in the Pathology Department at Cambridge University, envisaged a novel test that revoltionized the way blood group antibody/antigen reac-

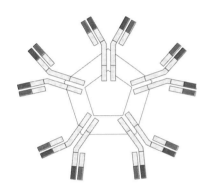

Direct agglutinating

Complete

Pentameric Ig

Multivalent

IgM

Disappearing

Non-agglutinating

Blocking

Incomplete

Indirect agglutinating

Monomeric Ig

Univalent

IgG

Fig. 8.3 Names associated with IgM and IgG

tions were (and still are) detected. The test, published by R.R.A. Coombs, A.E. Mourant and R.R. Race in the *Lancet* in 1945, is now well known as the "Coombs test". Coombs insisted that as he was only one of three authors, he preferred the name "antiglobulin test". In respect for the insight of Coombs, even staff in the laboratories of his co-authors, Mourant and Race, referred to the tile on which the antiglobulin test was performed as the "Coombs tile". However, out of respect for Coombs' own stated wishes, we will use the term "antiglobulin test" and not the "Coombs test" throughout this book.

When we visited Robin Coombs for this book, we found a modest, gentle man who insisted that his contribution was small; however, the test he conceived has and will continue to help millions. The test has had an immense impact; it detects the antibodies that were undetectable BC (before Coombs). It not only detects other antibodies causing transfusion reactions, HDN, and autoimmune hemolytic anemia, but also it is used to indicate the effectiveness of exchange transfusion. It can be used to estimate the amount of antibody in the child, and to quantify the amount of maternal antibody during pregnancy, which permits treatment to be evidence based. Moreover, by providing a sufficiently stringent way of detecting the vast majority of antigen/antibody combinations, it has enabled blood transfusion to become safer than driving home from the airport.

Robin Coombs (1921 – 2008)

Robin Coombs graduated in veterinary medicine from Edinburgh University and initially worked in Surrey, England in a veterinary laboratory although he never practiced as a vet. In 1943, he joined the Pathology Department at Cambridge University where he began work on a doctorate that he completed in 1947. He enjoyed the support of Professor "Daddy" Dean[1] (who had also backed Florey, winner of the Nobel Prize in 1945 for his role in the discovery of penicillin). At that time there was interest in the way physical things fitted together, expressed by the intriguingly simple interlocking blocks of Lego toys, invented by a Danish carpenter in 1934. At the molecular level, John Marrack in Dean's laboratory had proposed the lattice theory of precipitation. Another worker in Dean's laboratory had injected rabbits with human plasma to make anti-human globulin. Thus, Coombs possessed the building

1. **Henry Roy Dean (1879-1961)**
In 1904, Dean qualified at St. Thomas's Hospital, London. From 1922-1961, he was Professor of Pathology. "Daddy" Dean was loved and respected because he imparted unusual excitement when he taught. He conveyed his enthusiasm for pathology but especially for immunology, which at the time was an obscure corner of medicine. As Coombs recalled, he was appointed to the Chair in 1922, before mandatory retirement, and lectured into the 1950s when his slight unsteadiness on his feet added an element of suspense especially to those in the front row! Anyone who was taught by him, laughs warmly at the recollection of his innovative teaching. He was Master of Trinity Hall, Cambridge, 1955-1965. He died, still in the Chair, at the age of 82.

2. As important as Robin Coomb's discovery was, it amazes the authors of this book that when we visited the University Library in Cambridge in 2004, to get a copy of his PhD thesis entitled: "The Conglutinin and Sensitization Reactions" (half of which is devoted to his discovery and early use of the antiglobulin test) we were told: "We cannot let you view the thesis or copy it without a signature from the author. This requirement applies only to the first requester." It is hard to believe that in almost 60 years, no one had asked to read this breakthrough research in its original form. As we had Dr Coombs' signature, we obtained a copy of his thesis.

blocks needed to develop his revelation, the antiglobulin test.[2]

One day over coffee, Coombs met fellow researchers—Rob Race and Arthur Mourant, evacuees from London bombing—who told him that there were patients whose plasma contained non-agglutinating anti-D: Coombs was intrigued. Race gave him a plasma sample containing such an anti-D and, by using electrophoresis, Coombs demonstrated that the unseen anti-D was a globulin.

Soon after this, Coombs was on a train traveling from London to Cambridge trying to read some papers about immunology by Erhlich, in German. However, as the lighting and his German were poor, he closed his eyes and pondered why the non-agglutinating anti-D could not be detected on red cells. His inspiration was that if there was an antibody directed against the "blocking, incomplete" antibody on the red cells, the cells would agglutinate. Eureka!

Testing his hypothesis

The next day in Daddy Dean's laboratory, Coombs obtained some anti-human globulin, which had been made to study the optimal proportions of reagents for precipitation tests. Although this "anti-human globulin" (or anti-antibody) was crude, it worked well enough to show Coombs, Race, and Mourant that the principle was sound and they had a relatively simple test to detect non-agglutinating antibodies. They injected human globulin into rabbits and produced a more potent anti-antibody. Like other antibodies made in animals, this reagent had to be adsorbed to remove the unwanted anti-species antibodies (just like the absorptions that Landsteiner and Levine had done to prepare anti-M and anti-N). To accomplish this, Coombs used AB, D+ red cells. In the words of Coombs, "We tried it—and it worked—it worked well!" Fig. 8.4 depicts the principle of the antiglobulin test.

In 1945, Coombs, Mourant, and Race reported their landmark test. Unequivocally and reliably, they could detect incomplete antibodies. They followed their initial brief report with a more detailed account, but just as the page proofs were ready to be returned to the publisher, Arthur Mourant, an avid reader, became aware of a paper, published 37 years earlier (in 1908) by Carlo Moreschi , which described the same concept and had been referenced by Landsteiner. Moreschi had described a method to agglutinate a non-agglutinating antibody to typhoid bacteria by adding anti-goat antibody. Coombs always acknowledged Moreschi's priority.

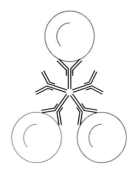

Direct agglutination

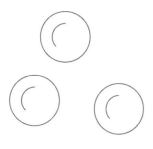

Sensitization

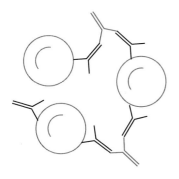

Indirect agglutination

Fig. 8.4 Principle of the antiglobulin test compared to the direct agglutination test. The anti-globulin reagent (red) acts as a bridge between any IgG molecules attached to the red cells, causing indirect agglutination.

He gave a lecture in Rome in 1953 entitled: "Moreschi and some recent developments in agglutination." Coombs told us that the antiglobulin test may turn out to be of lesser significance than his recent work attributing cot deaths to an anaphylactic reaction to inhaled milk proteins. Coombs had a life long interest in allergy, together with P.G.H. Gell, he developed the fourfold classification of immune response to tissue injury.

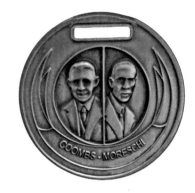

Fig 8.5 Robin Coombs/Carlo Moreschi South African National Blood Service Medal

Good news travels fast

The new antiglobulin test was a huge success. Race and Mourant collected blood samples from mothers of babies suspected of having HDN. They detected anti-D in a majority. In the minority of samples, they detected antibodies with other specificities.

Workers in blood banking are collegiate and friendly; thus, good news spread quickly throughout the world and the new invaluable test was ubiquitous within months. As will be described in the next two chapters, this led to the detection of many antibodies.

Chapter 9

Many More Antigens Revealed

Nobody sees a flower – really – it is so small – we haven't
time – and to see takes time.

—Georgia O'Keefe.

1. R.A. Fisher was an experimentalist,
statistician, geneticist, and eugenicist.
He was inventive, rigorous, passion-
ate, and feisty. He invented maximum
likelihood analysis and the analysis
of variance, for which the F statistic
was so named in his honor by George
Snedecor. When testing the null
hypothesis he reccomended that the
population means are the same in all
experimental classes. Fisher explained
the evolution of dominance thus:

The theory that disadvantageous genes are maintained in
all species by rare mutations,
the frequency of each (generally somewhat low) being such

The antiglobulin test led to the discovery of a vast variety of blood
groups; far more than could have been imagined by even the most
optimistic person. Blood group antigens are carried by a variety of
different molecules on the surface of the red cell that provoke the
production of antibodies. Without the presence of an antibody, the
antigen remains undetected. The antiglobulin test was a requirement
for the detection of many antibodies; especially IgG.

Within five years of the development of the antiglobulin test, a
very different facilitator of research appeared; Robert Race and Ruth
Sanger published the first edition of *Blood Groups in Man* (1950),
with a foreword by R.A. Fisher.[1] It was a model of clarity, impartial-
ity, accuracy, and a complete survey of the entire field. They described
current developments, predicted the future, and were generous with
praise.

Key investigators readily shared plasma and red cells with Race
and Sanger, thereby facilitating the identification of new blood groups
as soon they were detected. Investigators typed blood from staff members, then, as needed, they collected blood from staff whose red cells
expressed the desired combination of antigens and compiled antibody
identification panels. Some staff members were more popular than
others and were bled rather frequently. Group O was the preferred
blood type so they could be tested with plasma from all people. Reactivity could now be detected by the indirect agglutination test (antiglobulin test) as well as by the direct agglutination test (Fig. 8.4).
With these 'antibody identification panels', investigators could not
only identify known antibodies but could also quickly recognize a
new pattern of reactivity in plasma from a mother whose baby had
HDN or from a patient who had a transfusion reaction (Fig. 9.1).

Patient Name:_____   Date:_____

Donor	Pheno	D	C	E	c	e	M	N	S	s	P1	Le^a	Le^b	Lu^a	Lu^b	K	k	Kp^a	Js^a	Js^b	Fy^a	Fy^b	Jk^a	Jk^b	Xg^a	Sex	Direct	Indirect
1	R1R1	+	+	0	0	+	+	0	0	+	+	0	+	0	+	0	+	0	0	+	+	0	0	+	+	F	0	3+
2	R1R1	+	+	0	0	+	0	+	+	+	+	0	0	0	+	+	0	0	0	+	0	+	+	0	+	M	0	3+
3	R1R1	+	+	0	0	+	+	+	+	0	+	0	+	0	+	0	+	0	0	+	0	+	0	+	+	M	0	3+
4	R2R2	+	0	+	+	0	0	+	0	+	+	0	+	0	+	0	+	0	0	+	0	+	0	+	+	M	0	3+
5	R2R2	+	0	+	+	0	+	0	0	0	0	+	0	+	0	+	0	0	0	+	0	+	0	+	+	F	0	3+
6	R2r	+	0	+	+	+	0	+	0	0	+	+	0	+	+	0	+	0	0	0	0	+	+	+	+	F	1+	3+
7	R1r	+	+	0	+	+	+	+	+	+	+	0	+	0	+	+	+	0	0	+	+	0	+	0	+	M	0	3+
8	Ro	+	0	0	+	+	+	+	+	+	0	0	0	+	0	+	0	+	+	0	0	+	0	+	F	0	3+
9	r'r	0	+	0	+	+	+	+	0	+	+	0	0	0	+	0	+	0	0	+	+	+	0	0	0	M	0	0
10	rr	0	0	0	+	+	+	+	0	+	+	0	+	0	+	0	+	0	0	+	+	0	+	+	+	F	0	0
11	rr	0	0	0	+	+	+	+	+	0	+	0	+	0	+	0	+	0	0	+	0	0	0	+	+	F	0	0
12	rr	0	0	0	+	+	+	+	0	+	+	+	0	0	+	+	0	0	0	+	+	0	+	0	+	M	1+	1+
13	r'r	0	+	0	+	+	0	+	0	+	+	0	+	0	+	0	+	0	0	+	0	+	0	+	0	F	1+	1+
14	r"r	0	0	+	+	+	+	+	+	+	+	0	0	0	+	0	+	0	0	+	+	0	+	+	+	F	0	0

Fig. 9.1 A typical antibody identification panel that might be used today. The panel shows 14 red cell samples that have been typed for numerous blood group antigens. Reactivity for an antibody that agglutinates red cells by the direct agglutination test (anti-Le^a) is shown. The anti-Le^a is also detected by the antiglobulin test, which also reveals an anti-D.

A plethora of antibodies

One such antibody, which had been hypothesized by Fisher was anti-e. The antigen with which it reacted, e, is antithetical to the E antigen. The antithetical relationship was shown by family studies: all E− red cells were e+ and all e− red cells were E+. The family studies also showed that E and e antigens were inherited according to Mendel's rules. Anti-e was not reactive by direct agglutination; its detection had to await the antiglobulin test. The first reported example was found in the plasma from a multiply transfused patient. Like the other Rh antibodies, anti-e can cause HDN and transfusion reactions.

Among the 15 blood samples from mothers and babies with HDN that had been collected by Coombs, Race, and Mourant, there was one that was not anti-D. The red cells from the baby were shown to be coated with an antibody. Plasma from the mother did not agglutinate with any of 13 red cell samples typed for the known Rh antigens (D, C, c, E, and e), but did agglutinate red cells from the ABO-compatible father. This antibody reacted with 7% of random samples from Europeans. It was the second antibody specificity to be identified by the antiglobulin test. The antibody was named anti-Kell after the parents, Mr and Mrs Kelleher, and the antigen it recognized was initially called Kell. Today this antigen is more correctly called K, while the system of related antigens is called Kell (see Chapter 10).

Later in 1946, the same year Kell was discovered, an antibody that was clearly related to, but different from, anti-C was found in a patient who had been transfused numerous times. The antigen was called C^W—"C" because of the association with the

that the elimination by natural selection just balances fresh accretions by mutation; that similar mutations though rare events have occurred regularly in the past, often for enormous periods; that in this situation natural selection will constantly favor modifying factors tending to render each type of heterozygote more normal, or in other words to render the disadvantageous mutant more recessive; and that such recessive genes, though each rare compared with its normal allelomorph, exist in great numbers in different parts of the germ plasm. This theory, although strenuously combatted by Prof. Sewall Wright, appears now to be found generally acceptable.

Wright explained:

In 1929 I questioned R.A. Fisher's theory that the prevailing dominance of wild-type genes over deleterious mutations (of which even the heterozygotes were rare in nature) was due to natural selection of specific modifiers of these heterozygotes (selection pressure of the order of 10^{-6} as we both agreed). I maintain that the phenomenon could be explained more plausibly as a byproduct of selection of modifiers of the abundant wild-type homozygotes, reflecting the dosage-response curve of an enzymatic reaction limited by the rate of production of its substrate. Discussion got nowhere because of persistent misrepresentation of my hypothesis by Fisher and his associates. The great achievement of Beadle and Tatum in the 1940s was to correlate systematically steps in the basic metabolic reactions with genes, and in some cases demonstrate enzyme differences.

Fisher's strong belief in selection dominated much of his thinking. He showed how heterozygous advantage sustains balanced polymorphisms. He measured natural selection, and in 1930 suggested that it was the likely cause of the blood group distributions, with perhaps malaria or yellow fever as the selective factors, and indeed malaria has been shown to influence ABO group prevalence in Africa.

In 1935, Fisher persuaded the Medical Research Council to establish

C antigen, and "W" from "Willis", the last name of the person whose red cells expressed the antigen that stimulated the anti-C^W in the patient.

So, by the end of 1946, antithetical blood group antigens had been named using a variety of methods:

(a) a single upper case letter (e.g., A/B/O; M/N),

(b) an upper and a lower case letter (e.g., C/c; E/e),

(c) an upper case letter, a lower case letter, and an upper case letter with a superscript upper case letter (e.g., C/c/C^W),

(d) an upper case and a lower case letter with superscript "a" or "b" (e.g., Lu^a/Lu^b, Le^a/Le^b).

Further creative names were yet to come.

For twenty years after their discovery, M and N remained uncomplicated, and apparently complete. However, this phase of simplicity came to an end when plasma from a patient who was known to have anti-D was shown to contain an additional antibody that gave reactions different from any previously described. The plasma was investigated in 1947 by Bob Walsh at the New South Wales Blood Transfusion Service, Sydney, Australia. He sent a sample to Race and his Australian assistant, Ruth Sanger, at the Blood Group Research Unit in the Lister Institute, Chelsea, London. The relationship of the new antibody to M and N was revealed by using a mathematical tool, the 2 x 2 table. The prevalence of the new antigen was different among the three MN types (M+N−, M+N+, M−N+); more than two-thirds of M+ people were positive while only about one-third of N+ people were positive.

This relationship of the new antigen to M and N was revealed by Sanger while Race was on vacation. When he returned to work, he was so delighted that he threatened to take more holidays! Race and Sanger chose the name "S" after "Sydney"; the city from which both the sample containing anti-S and Ruth Sanger hailed.

After testing 1,419 red cell samples with anti-M, anti-N, and anti-S, Fisher calculated the gene frequencies. Given the linkage disequilibrium between S and M and N antigens (e.g., a much higher number of S+ red cells were M+ than M−), he surmised that an antigen antithetical to S existed and when found it would be called s. Indeed, in 1951 anti-s was found in the plasma of a mother whose second child was severely affected with HDN.

In 1949, an antibody was found in the plasma of a woman whose baby had mild HDN. The antibody agglutinated red cells

2 x 2 Contingency Tables

Karl Pearson ran the Department of Applied Statistics while being the first to hold the Galton Chair of Eugenics at University College, London. He championed statistics, he coined the term standard deviation, and he developed the chi-square method to test the significance of the differences between two or more sets of data, which he called a "2 x 2 contingency table".

R.A. Fisher, who succeeded Pearson in the Galton Chair, adapted his contingency tables for the analysis of small sample numbers. The test is known as "Fisher's exact test". Fisher devised the test following a comment from Muriel Bristol, a worker at Rothamsted Agricultural Experiment Station, who "declares that by tasting a cup of tea made with milk, she can discriminate whether the milk or the tea infusion was first added to the cup."

Fisher tested her claim by mixing eight cups of tea, four in one way and four in the other, and presenting them to her for judgment in a random order, and then he performed his exact test. Fisher does not give the results—perhaps because she actually could distinguish the order in which the milk and tea were added!

Fisher's reasoning can be applied to the identification of antibodies. Suppose only three K+ and two K– group O red cell samples are tested, and the unknown plasma agglutinates the three K+ samples but not the two K– samples. This would seem proof of the presence of anti-K but it is not adequate proof. According to Fisher's exact test, the probability of getting such a distribution by chance alone is 1 in 10:

Table 9.1 2 x 2 Contingency Table for K

	Known cells		Totals
	K+	K–	
Unknown plasma positive	3	0	= 3
Unknown plasma negative	0	2	= 2
Totals	3	2	= 5

Probability (p) = [(3!x2!x2!x3!) ÷ 5!] x (1 ÷ 3!x2!x0!x0!) = 1 in 10. (Factorial 3, or 3!, for example = 3 x 2 x 1; and factorial 0, 0!, surprisingly is 1, not 0).

When investigating a new antibody specificity, Race and Sanger "did not get excited until a probability of 1 in 100 was achieved". In the identification of familiar antibodies they were "usually satisfied with a probability of 1 in 40 or so".

a blood-group research laboratory that soon recruited a young medical assistant, Robert Race. In 1940, Janet Vaughan, head of the NW London blood depot, discovered that men and women had different ABO frequencies. Fisher attributed this to male migration. In 1943, Fisher predicted the genetics of Rh brilliantly, and his hypotheses have been confirmed, except that three closely linked genes were involved.

He failed to recognize the ease with which observer bias overcomes the best analysis. Fisher was addicted to tobacco and opposed Richard Doll and Bradford Hill's demonstration that smoking was carcinogenic. He was also addicted to an upper class English life style and opposed UNESCO's race blindness. As a eugenicist, he had 9 children, of whom one was an Rh– daughter who agreed to marry her prospective husband if and only if he was also Rh–. He was.

Fisher will be remembered as the person who more than anyone founded twentieth century statistics as a science. He will also be remembered as the person whose contribution to evolutionary biology was as important as that of Haldane and Wright.

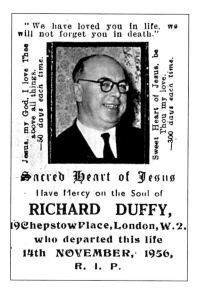

"We have loved you in life, we will not forget you in death."

Jesus, my God, I love Thee above all things. —50 days each time.

Sweet Heart of Jesus, be Thou my love. —300 days each time.

Sacred Heart of Jesus

Have Mercy on the Soul of

RICHARD DUFFY,

19 Chepstow Place, London, W. 2.

who departed this life

14th NOVEMBER, 1956,

R. I. P.

Fig. 9.2 Mr Richard Duffy

from most people, but did not agglutinate red cells from the mother or from five of 2,500 blood samples tested. All six non-reactive samples were K+. The antigen was named Cellano, an anagram of the woman's last name (Nocella). When its antithetical relationship to K was proven, the antigen was renamed k.

In 1950, a pattern of reactions was observed that was clearly different from any of the established blood groups. The antibody was found in the plasma of a hemophiliac patient, Mr Duffy, who had a mild transfusion reaction after a series of transfusions received over the previous 20 years. To avoid confusion with the C-D-E (Rh), symbols, instead of the letter D, the symbol Fy, from the last two letters of Mr Duffy's name, was selected.

In 1951, in addition to anti-s, several other new antibodies were described, including anti-Tj^a, anti-Jk^a, anti-Fy^b, and anti-Mi^a. Anti-Tj^a (now called anti-PP1P^k) was encountered in plasma from a woman with gastric cancer. It agglutinated red cells from 3,000 group O donors but not red cells from the donor herself or three of her brothers and sisters. This is an example of a so-called "public", or high prevalence, antigen. Jk^a was named in honor of Mr and Mrs Kidd, who brought this antigen to light. The mother, Mrs Kidd, made an antibody to an antigen on her husband's red cells. Their sixth son, John, had HDN, maybe due to the new antibody and/or to anti-K, which was also present in the maternal plasma. As the letter K had already been used, the new antigen was named Jk^a using the initials of this offspring, John Kidd. Another antigen, named Fy^b, because it was antithetical to Fy^a, was detected by an antibody in the plasma of a woman from Berlin during routine post-natal examination following the birth of her third child. Although none of her children had HDN, the pregnancies had to have elicited production of the antibody because the mother had not been transfused. The antithetical relationship of the new antigen to Fy^a was shown by using Fisher's 2 x 2 test. Initially, samples from 59 donors of known Fy^a type were tested, giving a probability of getting the same results by chance of 1 in 167.

Table 9.2 2 x 2 Contingency Table for Fy^a

	Fy(+)	Fy(a–)
Unknown plasma +	28	20
Unknown plasma –	11	0

The last antibody to be reported in 1951 was anti-Mi[a]. This antibody was detected in the plasma from Mrs Miltenberger after she gave birth to a baby with HDN. This antibody detected a "private" or low prevalence antigen. Over several years, when other related antibodies and antigens were found, they formed a subsystem of the MNS system named "Miltenberger". Once this subsystem evolved into eleven antigens, the name was declared obsolete and a terminology based on the name of the glycoprotein that carries the MNS antigens was introduced.

In 1952, the plasma of a patient who had a transfusion reaction was tested against red cells from 10,000 group O donors. It agglutinated red cells from all except the red cells from the antibody producer and from four of the donors. The antibody, anti-Vel was named after this patient.

In 1953, four more antigens were demonstrated: f in the Rh system, which had been originally thought to be antithetical to D but was later shown to be an antigen formed by the interaction of c and e antigens, while Jk[b], the antigen antithetical to Jk[a], disclosed itself when anti-Jk[b] was found in the plasma of a woman who had had a reaction to her second transfusion. This new antigen was shown to be antithetical to Jk[a] by using Fisher's 2 x 2 test. Samples from 98 donors of known Jk[a] type were tested, giving a probability of getting the same results by chance an impressive 1 in 14,129.

Table 9.3 2 x 2 Contingency Table for Jk[a]

	Jk(+)	Jk(a–)
Unknown plasma +	44	19
Unknown plasma –	35	0

The antigen detected by yet another antibody was named U from its almost universal distribution. Original tests revealed that anti-U agglutinated red cells from all white people tested, but not from twelve of 989 blacks. Later it was shown that all U– red cells are S–s–, but not all S–s– red cells are U–. This observation showed that U was part of the MNS system. Wr[a] was yet another antigen named after a family, the Wright family, who had a baby with HDN.

Availability of reagents

By the early 1950s, companies like Knickerbocker and Ortho sold pairs of typed red cell samples to detect antibodies to blood group antigens (antibody screening cells), panels of typed red cell samples (antibody identification panels, as in Fig. 9.1), and reagent antibodies. This provided laboratories in hospital transfusion services and blood donor centers with the necessary tools to detect and identify antibodies and to type red cells for antigens. Any sample with a new pattern of reactivity was sent to specialist reference laboratories. There followed an explosion of reports describing new antibodies.

By 1953, it was clear that antibodies to many different blood groups, the intragroup incompatibilities, were responsible for causing HDN and transfusion reactions. From 1953 to the publishing of this book in 2012, too many antibodies and antigens have been discovered to recount them all. But while Rh IgG was developed to prevent a D-negative woman from forming anti-D and thereby dramatically reducing the risk of HDN caused by anti-D, no such protective solution was, or indeed is, available against any of the other blood groups. However, knowledge of the clinical significance of a blood group antibody, the ability to identify these antibodies and to detect incompatibilities, has led to safe exchange transfusions to infants. This has resulted in a dramatic reduction in deaths from HDN.

The last animal-to-human transfusion

One antibody involves the last documented transfusion of animal blood to a human. The patient had a severe case of a cold autoimmune hemolytic anemia. Her plasma contained an autoantibody that reacted strongly at room temperature so that her red cells spontaneously agglutinated, which interfered with the determination of blood counts and her blood group. The autoantibody lysed her red cells in vivo, making her anemic. The patient suffered several hemolytic episodes that occurred after exposure to cold. One particularly bad episode happened in December after she worked all morning in an unheated office in Philadelphia. Another time, she had a transfusion reaction when transfused with blood that was cold. Subsequently, to avoid these reactions, during transfusions the blood and patient were kept warm. In tests against many red cell samples, one compatible donor was found. The antigen recognized by this antibody was named "I" to emphasize the high degree of individuality of red cells that did not react at room temperature. At 4°C, the patient's anti-I reacted even when her plasma was diluted 1 in 400,000! The patient was referred to Dr A.S. Wiener in New York. As compatible donors were scarce, he tested the patient's plasma against red cells from various animals. Red cells from rabbit, rhesus monkey, sheep, horse, and cow were agglutinated. However, as the agglutination of red cells from cows was the weakest, he decided to transfuse the patient with bovine red cells; (we think without the patient's informed consent). Blood was collected from the jugular vein of a previously tested, healthy cow. The red cells were washed seven times to remove the bovine plasma and 50 mL of a 50% suspension were injected slowly into a vein. Remarkably, there was no immediate reaction. However, after 15 minutes, the "patient suddenly became extremely apprehensive, had a sense of impending doom, complained of difficulty in breathing, and asked for oxygen". Wiener documented there was "no abnormality in heart sounds or respirations to account for her complaints". Nonetheless, oxygen was administered and epinephrine hydrochloride was injected subcutaneously. Fortunately, the patient's complaints quickly subsided but as Wiener reported in 1956: "This reaction discouraged us from further attempts at transfusion of bovine red cells."

Grand Rapids makes history with Mr And

In 1962, during crossmatching for a blood transfusion in a hospital in Grand Rapids, Michigan, a fascinating new antibody was found in the plasma of Mr And. This patient had been transfused many times for severe nosebleeds due to familial telangiectasia. One or more of these transfusions had stimulated him to produce an antibody that did not recognize any of the known blood group antigens. A blood sample, together with the results of testing his family, was sent to Race and Sanger, who spotted that the antigen occurred twice as often in females as in males, which is expected in X-linked dominant inheritance. They added:

> A rather neat confirmation of the X-linkage of a character such as Xg is provided by XO Turner females having the male distribution of the antigen.

It was not until 1688 that color blindness was recognized by Robert Boyle. Over the previous thousand millennia, no one had noticed that one man in twelve had difficulty recognizing when an apple or a tobacco leaf was ripe. It took another two centuries to recognize that color blindness has a pattern of male to female to male inheritance, that is, the gene is an X-linked recessive. In contrast, within minutes of receiving the test results on Mr And's blood and his family, Race and Sanger spotted that the antigen detected by the antibody in his plasma was encoded by a gene located on the X chromosome. Blood samples from more families were tested and, one after the other showed that inheritance of the antigen obeyed the rules for X-linked dominant inheritance. This was the first blood group antigen discovered to be on the X-chromosome, and was named Xg^a, "X" for the chromosome, and "g" for "Grand Rapids". This X-linked red cell antigen was immediately seen to have possible use as a marker to measure linkage, to observe meiosis, and to observe the stage at which X-chromosome abnormalities and aneuploidies arose. Mary Lyon (Fig. 9.3) predicted that around the 16th day of embryogenesis one or other of the two X chromosomes in each somatic cell was randomly inactivated, generating an adult that would be a patchwork of cells, some with an active X and others with an inactive X. Thanks to Mr And's anti-Xg^a, the two populations of red cells could be identified if they existed, but they did not.

Mary Lyon drew her inspiration from the mosaic color pattern in mice heterozygous for an X-linked fur melanin gene. If one of the two X chromosomes was inactivated, then any one lineage of cells derived from that cell would receive an inactivated gene

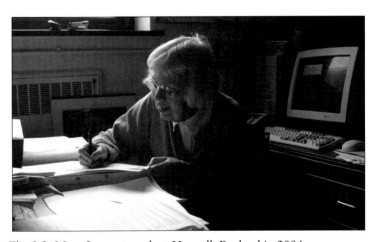

Fig. 9.3 Mary Lyon at work at Harwell, England in 2004

(maternally or paternally derived). In honor of Mary Lyon, this now proven process is called "lyonization." Unlike most genes on the X chromosome, Xg^a escaped lyonization—no mosaicism for Xg^a has been demonstrated. In 1981, another blood group antigen, CD99, was found which also escapes lyonization and is phenotypically related to Xg^a, and is encoded by a gene in the pseudoautosomal regions on the short arm of X and Y chromosomes. It led to the discovery of a region on both X and Y in which pairing and crossing-over occur.

Other laboratories copied Race and Sanger's practice of listing sex of donors used to constitute the antibody identification panels (Fig. 9.1)—just in case another sex-linked blood group antigen should show up. One did: Kx.

The original anti-Kx was found in a mixture of antibodies in the plasma of a Dutch boy, Claas, which reacted with all red cells tested, except his own. This reactivity was called anti-KL. As red cells from Claas had a weak expression of the Kell antigens, k and Kp^b, an association with Kell was assumed. The letter "K" likely comes from this observation and "L" because it was the next letter in the alphabet. The antibody was removed from plasma by adsorption onto red cells of chosen types and then eluted to recover the separated antibody specificities. The eluted preparations were tested with a selected panel of red cells and two different patterns of agglutination were obtained. The antibody in one eluate was called anti-Km and in the other, anti-Kx. Anti-Km ("m" as the next letter in the alphabet and for "modified") failed to agglutinate red cells that lacked all Kell antigens (the so-called Kell$_{null}$ phenotype) and those with a weak expression of Kell antigens (from Claas and from Hugh McLeod, a Harvard dental student). In contrast, anti-Kx strongly agglutinated Kell$_{null}$ red cells, weakly agglutinated red cells of common Kell type, and did not agglutinate red cells from Claas or Hugh McLeod. Red cells of this type are said to have the McLeod phenotype (see Chapter 15). Relatives of Claas and Hugh McLeod with red cells having the McLeod phenotype had pedigrees that were consistent with X-linked recessive inheritance, like hemophilia. Hence the name "Kx" was coined for the antigen lacking from red cells with the McLeod phenotype (K from the association with Kell antigens and x from X-linkage).

Compatibility testing

As we have explained, people who are transfused or pregnant may be exposed to a foreign blood group antigen and thus make antibodies to it or them. At each exposure there is a possibility that additional antibodies will be made. The antibodies can be to any of the multitude of antigens, and in any combination. A patient with sickle cell disease, thalassemia, aplastic anemia, or chronic bleeding due to hemophilia or hereditary telangiectasia may require repeated transfusions. Because of the vast array of different combinations of foreign antigens on red cells, receiving blood almost always introduces foreign antigens and these antigens trigger antibody production in the recipient's plasma. Once antibodies have been produced, the next exposure to blood with the triggering antigen may cause a transfusion reaction. Thus, these patients have special needs with regard to donor blood and it is important to select and transfuse red cells that lack antigens corresponding to the antibodies in the patient's plasma.

Blood is always matched for ABO. While all patients can receive blood from donors with the same ABO blood group, only some can also receive blood from certain other ABO blood groups. As group O has neither A nor B antigens, group O blood can be safely transfused to group O patients (identical match), as well as to A, B, and AB patients (compatible match). On the other hand, group O patients have anti-A and anti-B in their plasma and can only receive group O red cells; they cannot receive blood from group A, B, or AB donors.

Table. 9.4 Cross testing ABO groups in patients and donors

Blood Type of Donor	Blood Type of Patient			
	O	A	B	AB
O	Identical	Compatible	Compatible	Compatible
A	Incompatible	Identical	Incompatible	Compatible
B	Incompatible	Incompatible	Identical	Compatible
AB	Incompatible	Incompatible	Incompatible	Identical

Before each transfusion, blood is also tested to ensure a match to all other blood group antigens. Plasma from a patient is tested against reagent red cells to detect antibody activity. If an antibody is detected, it is identified using a reagent panel of red cells (as in Fig. 9.1). If more than one antibody is present in the plasma, the approach used to identify them all can become complex and time consuming, and is beyond the scope of this book. If an antibody is identified, red cells from the patient are tested to confirm they lack the corresponding antigen. To prevent a transfusion reaction, donor red cells selected for transfusion should lack antigens corresponding to antibodies in the patient's plasma. This applies for the rest of the life of the patient.

Locating compatible blood

Blood for transfusion that is matched for ABO and Rh only, as in the majority of transfusions, is available from the inventory of blood components stored at the hospital. When the matching needs to be more precise, blood may be available from the inventory at the hospital, but is more likely obtained from the inventory at the donor center that supplies the hospital. Donor centers have a larger inventory of antigen-negative red cell components than does any given hospital. The antigen-negative inventory includes many different combinations of antigen negativity that can be liquid (stored in a refrigerator) and ready for immediate shipment to the hospital when the patient needs a blood transfusion, or may be stored frozen. Just like food products, frozen blood lasts years longer than the liquid blood. A liquid red cell component has a shelf-life of weeks, while that of a frozen component has a shelf-life of years.

Rarely, a patient's plasma contains an antibody or antibodies that makes it difficult to find suitable antigen-negative blood for transfusion. When this happens, the donor center will contact either a larger donor center or, more likely, the national Rare Donor Registry. In extremely rare cases, it may be necessary to access the International Rare Donor Panel. The network in place ensures that a patient who needs blood will get it. Some patients give their own (autologous) blood.

Too many names

By 1980, 232 antigens had been described. Their sheer number, let alone their colorful and varied names, were somewhat overwhelming and it was clear that a system was needed to give some order to the alphabet soup. By this time, the value of computer databases had been accepted. Thus, the International Society of Blood Transfusion (ISBT) formed a working party to develop a scheme for naming blood group antigens that is "both eye and machine readable, and in keeping with the genetic basis of blood groups". The scheme that was developed is still in use today.

Chapter 10

Blood Group Systems and Beyond

> You may call a spade a spade, but I will call it whatever
> I please.
>
> —George Bernard Shaw

We hesitated to quote Shaw, who thought of spades as sturdy garden tools or as the highest suit in bridge. At that time, the word
had not yet acquired its slang derogatory meaning. It makes our
point that everyday words can be ambiguous and have influence
beyond their mere label. In 1953, the philosopher John Wisdom
made a similar point in responding to a review of his recent book in
the *New Statesman* by a colleague at Reading University, who said
it was a pity that he did not explain his own philosophy. Wisdom
demonstrated his view that philosophical problems were merely
linguistic entanglements by his reply:

> Can you take a good strong wooden box containing two
> parrots and later take out 22 parrots all talking like human
> beings?

In his next lecture he explained that as soon as the words were
defined, paradoxes and philosophies disappear, How much later?
Was the box a conjuring trick with a trap-door? Did the parrots
talk English or just repeat sounds? Paradoxes and imprecision are
amusing pabulum to philosophers but are unacceptable perils to
blood bankers. The confusing multiplicity of antigen names had to
be replaced, to ensure that the names were clear and distinct.

Historically, antigens were usually named after either the
first person whose red cells carried the antigen, or the first person whose plasma contained the antibody. In the early literature,
names were freely used in publications; nowadays, the name of
a proband cannot be used in the name of an antigen without her
or his permission. The resultant hodgepodge of names made con-

versation awkward. As there were no rules or oversight, the same antibody specificity could be found by different workers, and given different names. There was a need for order.

The profusion of different names was highly undesirable: data stored was sometimes intelligible only to the workers storing them, and it impeded interchange of information, which is a valuable asset of an electronic database. To overcome this problem, the International Society of Blood Transfusion (ISBT) Working Party on Automation and Data Processing recommended the formation of a Working Party on Terminology for Red Cell Surface Antigens. This Working Party made order out of the chaos.

Formation of ISBT working party on terminology for red cell surface antigens

A group of 32 eminent international investigators in the field of blood groups attended the inaugural meeting in Montreal in 1980. The Working Party followed rules of the human gene nomenclature group, and agreed henceforth to eliminate Greek letters, superscripts and subscripts, and to use only capital letters of the Roman alphabet, and Arabic numerals to name blood group antigens. A high priority of the Working Party was to assign a number for each blood group antigen—for use in databases—in addition to, not replacement for, the more easily remembered historical names.

BLOOD GROUP SYSTEMS

A blood group system is a discrete genetic entity under the control of a single gene or a cluster of two (Rh, Chido/Rodgers systems) or three (MNS system) closely-related homologous genes. The different antigens within a system are encoded by alternative forms of the gene. Until the late 1980s, proof that an antigen was under the control of a gene was based on family studies. These studies demonstrated the antithetical relationship between antigens, e.g. K and k. Linkage provided evidence that genes were or were not separate on a chromosome and thus were or were not accepted for inclusion within a blood group system, e.g. MN and Ss were part of the same system. When an antibody failed to react with pertinent "null phenotype" red cells, the new antigen was placed in that blood group system.

Based on the information available, in 1990 the Working Party allocated 157 blood group antigens to 19 blood group systems and developed symbols for each system. Antigens that did not belong in a blood group system, because their controlling genes were not known, were placed into "Collections" of 35 antigens with a serological, biochemical, or genetic relationship, a series of 37 uncommon antigens (less than 1% in most populations studied), or a series of 13 common antigens (more than 90% in most populations studied). The Working Party also provided guidelines for establishing a new blood group system, adding a new antigen into an established system, obtaining a new ISBT number, and naming novel antigens.

A symbol for a newly described antigen must consist of three to six capital letters and must not duplicate, alphabetically or phonetically, any current or obsolete symbols for blood groups or related disciplines. Examples of antigens named in this way are DAK, GUTI, HAG, JAL, KREP, MARS, MINY, RAZ, STAR, STEM, TSEN, TOU, VLAN, each name being derived from the name of each proband. DANE was named after the antigen found on red cells from members of four Danish families; and FPTT, was named after the "French Post Telegraph and Telecommunications" because several of the original probands worked and donated blood there. Names ENEP, ENEH, ENAV and ENDA were given to common antigens in the MNS system; "EN" was used because the antigens are carried on an important glycoprotein of the envelope of the red cell membrane.

Database numbers

The Working Party developed a classification whereby each antigen had a unique 6-digit number. The first 3 digits represented the system, and the second 3 digits represented the antigen within the system. Table 10.1 lists designations for each of the 30 blood group systems and some antigens. Each system has three names: a traditional name (e.g. Duffy) that is used for verbal communication and in publications; a symbol of upper case letters for use in a database (e.g. FY); and a 3-digit number, also for use in a database (e.g. 006). Each antigen also has three names: a traditional name (e.g. Fy^a) that is used for verbal communication and in publications; a symbol of upper case letters for use in a database (e.g. FY1); and a 3-digit number within its system, also for use in a database (e.g. 006001). These designations are still in use today. The number of antigens in each system ranges from 1 to more than 50 but, for the sake of brevity, only three are given for each system in Table 10.1.

Table 10.1 Current blood group systems and antigens

Traditional name	ISBT Symbol	System number	Antigen number			# of antigens
			001	**002**	**003**	
ABO	ABO	001	A	B	A,B	1 more
MNS	MNS	002	M	N	S	43 more
P	P1PK	003	P1	P^k		
Rh	RH	004	D	C	E	49 more
Lutheran	LU	005	Lu^a	Lu^b	Lu3	17 more
Kell	KEL	006	K	k	Kp^a	29 more
Lewis	LE	007	Le^a	Le^b	Le^{ab}	3 more
Duffy	FY	008	Fy^a	Fy^b	Fy3	2 more
Kidd	JK	009	Jk^a	Jk^b	Jk3	
Diego	DI	010	Di^a	Di^b	Wr^a	19 more
Yt	YT	011	Yt^a	Yt^b		
Xg	XG	012	Xg^a	CD99		
Scianna	SC	013	Sc1	Sc2	Sc3	4 more
Dombrock	DO	014	Do^a	Do^b	Gy^a	4 more
Colton	CO	015	Co^a	Co^b	Co3	1 more
Landsteiner-Wiener	LW	016	*			3
Chido-Rodgers	CH/RH	017	Ch1	Ch2	Ch3	6 more
H	H	018	H			
Kx	XK	019	Kx			
Gerbich	GE	020	**	Ge2	Ge3	8 more
Cromer	CROM	021	Cr^a	Tc^a	Tc^b	13 more
Knops	KN	022	Kn^a	Kn^b	McC^a	6 more
Indian	IN	023	In^a	In^b	INFI	1 more
Ok	OK	024	Ok^a	OKGV	OKGM	
Raph	RAPH	025	MER2			
John Milton Hagen	JMH	026	JMH	JMHK	JMHL	3 more
I	I	027	I			
Globoside	GLOB	028	P			
Gil	GIL	029	GIL			
RhAG	RHAG	030	Duclos	Ol^a	DSLK	

* Antigens in the LW (016) system were renamed and numbers 001 to 004 were made obsolete. There are three antigens in the LW blood group system.
** Ge1 antigen was declared obsolete when antibody and typed red cells were no longer available.

Summary of blood group systems

In addition to the 284 antigens in the current 30 blood group systems, there are, as of June 2010, 43 that are not yet placed in any blood group system; 17 antigens in seven Collections, 18 uncommon antigens, and 8 common antigens.

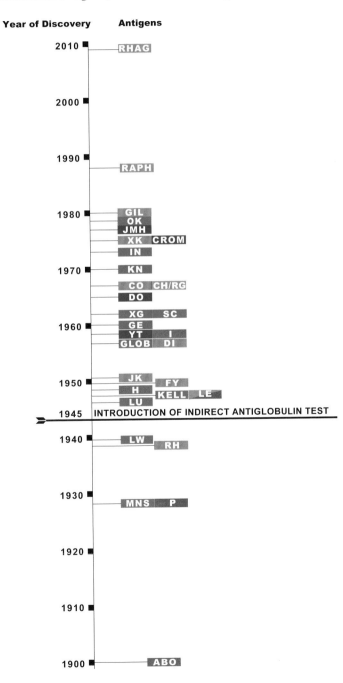

Fig. 10.1 Date of discovery or elucidation of the first antigen in each blood group systems. The color represents the type of red cell membrane component that carries the antigens in the system.

Table 10.2 A brief description of how each blood group system was named

Blood Group System	How System Was Named
ABO	First 2 letters of alphabet and O from "ohne", which is German for "without"
MNS	First found in immune rabbit plasma, with S from Sydney, Australia & Ruth Sanger
P	Next letter in alphabet after M, N, and O
Rh	Rhesus monkey red cells were used to stimulate anti-"Rh" in animals
Lutheran	Name of first donor who stimulated production of anti-Lu³; his name was Lutteran, but it was misread
Kell	Kelleher, the first family with HDN due to anti-K
Lewis	One of the two original donors in whom anti-Le³ was identified
Duffy	A hemophiliac who made the first anti-Fy³
Kidd	Name of first family with HDN due to anti-Jk³; "Jk" were the initials of the baby (John Kidd)
Diego	Name of first family, Mr and Mrs Diego from Venezuela, whose child had HDN due to anti-Di³
Yt	When the antibody to this high prevalence antigen was found, most letters in the patient's name (Cartwright) had been taken by other antigens. The authors thought "why not "T", then "why T", which became "Yt"
Xg	X for the X chromosome and "g" from Grand Rapids, where the patient, Mr And, was treated
Scianna	Family name of the first patient to make anti-Sc1 (originally called anti-Sm)
Dombrock	Family name of the first patient to make anti-Do³
Colton	Family name of the first patient to make anti-Co³. Should have been called "Calton", but the handwriting on the test tube was misread
Landsteiner-Wiener	In honor of Landsteiner and Wiener who made this antibody in animals after immunizing them with blood from rhesus monkey (originally called Rh)
Chido/Rodgers	First antibody producers of anti-Ch and anti-Rg
H	From heterogeneous, when it was shown that the fucose was common to the great majority of red cells irrespective of their ABO group
Kx	Kx was shown to be associated with the Kell blood group system but controlled by a gene on the X chromosome
Gerbich	Family name of one of three mothers, found at the same time, who made anti-Ge
Cromer	Family name of the first patient to make anti-Cr³
Knops	Family name of the first patient to make anti-Kn³
Indian	The first In(a+) people were from India
Ok	Derived from one of the names of the first patient, Ko from Japan, to make anti-Ok³
RAPH	Abbreviation of the first name of the first patient to make anti-MER2. The only antigen in this system retains the MER2 name as it was previously identified by a monoclonal antibody, MER2. "M" was derived from monoclonal and "ER" from Eleanor Roosevelt Hospital, the name of the institution that made the monoclonal antibody.
John Milton Hagen	Name of the first patient to make anti-JMH. Previously referred to as "Old Boys", because the original antibody producers were predominantly older men
I	I emphasizes the high degree of individuality of blood samples failing to react with a potent cold antibody
Globoside	Named after it was shown that the P antigen consists of the two terminal sugars (galactosamine-galatose) on globoside, which is a glycolipid
Gill	Abbreviation of family name of first patient to make anti-GIL
RhAG	Rh from the Rh system and AG for associated glycoprotein, which is required for expression of Rh antigens

Table 10.3 Examples of antigen names

Alphabetized Antigens		
A	AnWj	Auª
B	BARC	Beª
C	c	Co3
D	DAK	Diᵇ
E	e	Enª
f	Fyª	Fyᵇ
G	Ge2	Gyª
H	Hop	Hy
I	IFC	Inª
Jkª	JMH	Jsª
K	Kpª	Kx
Lan	Lu4	LWª
M	MAR	Mᵍ
N	NFLD	Noᵇ
Or	Okª	Olª
P1	Pᵏ	Prª
Rh29	Riv	Rd
S	Sc1	Sdª
Tcª	TSEN	Tar
U	Ulª	UMC
Vel	VS	Vw
WESª	Wrª	Wb
Xgª		
Ykª	Ytª	Ytᵇ
ZENA		

Over the years, blood group antigens have been designated by a variety of symbols: single letters (upper and lower case), two letters (one upper case; one lower case) with a superscript or number, a letter and a number, and three or four letters. Every letter of the alphabet (except Q) has been used at least once. Examples of antigen names are given in Table 10.3—note the variety. Although this has led to a somewhat cumbersome and awkward terminology, it is colorful, and each name has a story attached to it.

To introduce an element of logic in naming antigens, more recent names have started with the system symbol. Some examples are: KYO and KUCI, in the Kell (KEL) system with the other letters "YO" and "UCI" derived from the name of the proband; GEIS, the "GE" from the Gerbich (GE) system with "IS" derived from the proband's name; CENR and CEST, the "CE" comes from the RhCE protein of the Rh system with "NR" and "ST" derived from the names of the probands. Another antigen, in the Rh blood group system and also carried on the RhCE protein (CE), is named CEAG, with the "A" derived from the amino acid, arginine, associated with the common antigen, and "G" from the amino acid, glycine, which is present in the rare antithetical antigen-negative form of the RhCE protein (CEAG–).

Blood group antigens are expressed on proteins or carbohydrates in the red cell membrane. The red cell membrane consists of various proteins, lipids, and carbohydrates with different shapes, sizes, and textures.

We noticed that there are more Celtic names, especially in the early days, in our tables than one would expect. If some kind person could give the explanation (we do not have one), we will be happy to add it to the next edition of this book with attribution.

Chapter 11

Chromosomal Assignments

Cell and tissue, shell and bone, leaf and flower, are so many portions of matter, and it is in obedience to the laws of physics that their particles have been moved, moulded and conformed.

—D'Arcy Thompson

Early Chromosomes

Modern genetics rests on three major independent discoveries that were published less than twenty years apart in the mid nineteenth century. Charles Darwin discovered natural selection (1859), Gregor Mendel[1] discovered the laws of inheritance (1866) and Walther Flemming discovered chromosomes (1878). It was not until the twentieth century before they were dovetailed together. The term genetics was introduced by William Bateson in 1906, and the term gene was introduced by Wilhelm Johannsen in 1909.

J.B.S. Haldane and Julia Bell were the first to measure linkage of human genes—between hemophilia and color blindness—on the X chromosome. Today, all known genes can not only be confidently assigned to a chromosome but to their precise place on the chromosome. Once Tjio and Levan (1956), had established a good method for culturing and preparing chromosomes, the normal number of chromosomes of humans including the sex chromosomes, was shown to be 46 and not 48. At that time, chromosomes could be identified only by their overall length and the position of the centromere, which separates a short (petite, hence p) arm from a longer arm q [it is not clear whether "q" came from "queue" (French for tail) or because "q" was the next letter in the alphabet after "p"]. By squashing, boiling and staining them with carmine ascetic acid, Heitz and Bauer (1933), discovered giant chromosomes with light and dark bands, like a bar code. Theophilus Painter published the same finding, later that year (Fig. 11.1). When Larry Snyder, the professor of genetics at Ohio State University saw the paper, he excitedly showed it to his

1. GREGOR MENDEL (1822–1884), a Moravian monk, studied in Vienna from 1851–1853, but returned to Brünn (now Brno) in 1856 where he started his experiments on garden peas. He found that parental characteristics appeared in the offspring in definite ratios. He made hybrids of many thousands of pea plants, french beans, bush beans, and scarlet runner beans over many generations to confirm these ratios. In so doing, he discovered how traits are passed from parents to their offspring. He discovered the laws of inheritance.

Mendel presented his conclusions in 1865. They were ignored or unknown until 1900, when they were discovered "independently" by three botanists, and were then accepted universally, except by Marxists who considered the principles of Mendel-Morganism false and the hereditary

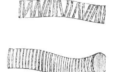

Fig. 11.1 Detailed drawing of Painter's salivary gland chromosome of *Drosophila* (1933)

student Charlie Cotterman, and they decided to share it with Mr. Muller who taught biology at the university.

> Snyder: We have come to show you a beautiful new finding of chromosomal banding patterns.
> Muller: It is beautiful, but it is not new.
> Snyder: Indeed it is new, it is in the current issue of the *Journal of Heredity*.
> Muller: However, I think there is an earlier report.

Fig. 11.2 E.G. Balbiani 1881 Giant banded chromosomes

Whereupon, he pulled from his shelf an 1881 article by Balbiani that showed banding patterns on salivary gland chromosomes of Chironomus (Fig. 11.2)

In Stockholm in 1968, Torbjorn Caspersson and others demonstrated that quinacrine mustard gave banding patterns on human metaphase chromosomes. This dye differentially stained euchromatic (genetically active) and heterochromatic (genetically inert) regions of chromosomes. Depending on the dye used, different banding patterns were obtained. The most common were Q-bands and G-bands resulting from staining with quinacrine and giemsa dyes respectively. Using these stains, each human chromosome possessed a unique pattern of bands that accurately distinguished one chromosome from another.

Chromosome banding

Bands are numbered using the centromere as the reference point. On diagrams, the short (p) arm is depicted above, and the long (q) arm is depicted below, the centromere. Moving from the centromere toward the ends, each band is numbered consecutively: the bands closest to the centromere were numbered as p1 or q1, the next p2 or q2, and so on. With greater resolution, each band contains subbands, which are also numbered consecutively. Further, each subband may be resolved into sub-sub-bands. Thus, the location of a gene can be given a precise "address". For example, the gene for ABO is located on chromosome 9 at q34.2 (Fig.11.3). The genetic

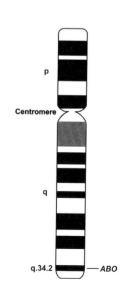

Fig. 11.3 Stylized chromosome 9

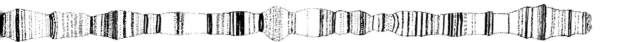

substance mythical.

Mendel concluded that inheritance is based upon pairs of particulate elements (now called genes) each of which determine specific traits. Offspring receive one or the other of each pair from each parent. Of each pair of elements acquired by the offspring, one is dominant and the other is recessive.

When both parents contribute a dominant element or when both parents contribute a recessive element the individual will be "pure" for that trait. If the parents contribute one dominant and one recessive, the individual will be a hybrid, but will look the same as the pure dominant. Mendel inferred the segregation and assortment of genes from the mathematical ratios of the observed phenotypes. Since these paired elements, whether dominant or recessive, are capable of separating, reappearing in their original form and pairing differently in later unions, they are obviously not contaminated or altered in any way in their passage from generation to generation.

If two or more pairs of elements are hybrids in a single plant, they assort independently in the formation of eggs and sperm.

Mendel used pea plants because they grow quickly and it is easy to see their different traits (e.g., purple or white flowers, yellow or green pods, long or short stems, round or wrinkled seeds). He discovered that traits show up in offspring without blending pa-

address is similar to a street address in which number 9 chromosome is represented by, say, 9th Street, whose eastern and western ends are separated by Fifth Avenue, just as the centromere separates the p and q arms. Thus, 9q34 corresponds to 9th street roughly three and a half blocks west of Fifth Avenue, and 34.2 corresponds to the house number in that block. Today, the Human Genome Project has generated even greater precision in an "address". Each nucleotide is identified with a RefSNP, or "rs", number. In the analogy above, the rs number relates to a certain window pane or even a brick in the house. For example, two SNPs in the A gene reside at rs7853989 and rs8176743.

Chromosomes consist of nucleotides

At the Rockefeller Institute in 1944, Oswald Avery, Maclyn Mc-Carty and Colin MacLeod demonstrated that deoxyribonucleic acid (DNA), not protein, could be the genetic material in pneumococci. Within 9 years the genetic instructions that determine our anatomy, physiology and perhaps even our thinking, was found to consist of a simple four-letter code embedded in DNA, that when coiled, wrapped in proteins and condensed, is recognized as a chromosome. The letters of the code are four simple organic nitrogenous bases: adenine, cytosine, guanine and thymine, abbreviated to A, C, G, and T. The order of these bases, called the sequence, has been determined for all human genes and is publicly available at the National Center for Biotechnology Information.

The human genome contains at least 3×10^9 bases and every cell in the body—except red cells, platelets and the lens—contains a complete copy, even though not all genes are active in all cells. These genes, which encode instructions, are passed with high fidelity from one generation to the next. However, occasionally a nucleotide change occurs, changing one base to another. A change in a base is called a single nucleotide polymorphism (SNP), and the two or more alternate forms of the gene are called alleles. In humans, there are millions of SNPs, but the process of such a change has only rarely been observed.

Blood groups and chromosomes

In 1968, R.P. Donahue, et al. made a tentative assignment of Duffy to chromosome 1, which was later shown to be correct, while Kidd was assigned to chromosome 21, which proved to be incorrect. Eloise Giblett (Elo) is remembered for an uncommon blood group antigen (ELO), for her authoritative book, *Genetic Markers in Human Blood* (1969), and for being a very nice person. Her book mentions the reports placing Duffy, Kidd and others on specific chromosomes, adding: "Much more evidence is needed to determine if these preliminary assignments are correct."

Using techniques available today (cloning, sequencing, and data from the Human Genome Project), each gene that encodes a blood group system has been assigned to a specific chromosome and given a precise location on that chromosome. Of the 30 blood group systems, 28 are on 14 of the 22 autosomes and 2—XG and XK—are on the X-chromosome (Fig. 11.4). Furthermore, many alleles have been sequenced.

Linkage of genes

Genes on different chromosomes, or those far apart on the same chromosome, segregate independently. Genes that are close together tend to segregate together unless there is crossing-over of chromosomes between the genes during meiosis—the extraordinary dance that the chromosomes perform when the pairs separate to make the sperm and egg (see Fig. 11.5). Except for part of the sex chromosomes, at meiosis every pair of chromosomes exchanges DNA rather like shuffling two packs of cards. If two cards are adjacent they are less likely to be separated in a shuffle than are two cards ten cards apart, which in turn are less likely to be separated than are two cards

rental characteristics.

Mendel's segregation principles hold true, and his postulated genes have been verified, first physically, then chemically. The gene occupies a very specific locus on a chromosome, and it may or may not encode or it may encode more than one product. One example that involves blood groups is the GYPC gene. If initiation occurs at the first AUG codon, glycophorin C (GPC) is encoded, but if initiation occurs at the second AUG codon, a shorter protein, glycophorin D (GPD) results.

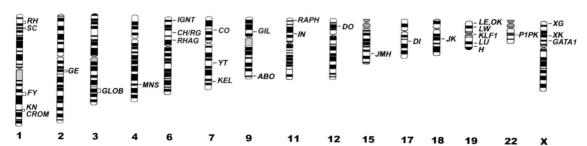

Fig. 11.4 Chromosomal locations of the genes encoding or influencing the expression of blood group antigens

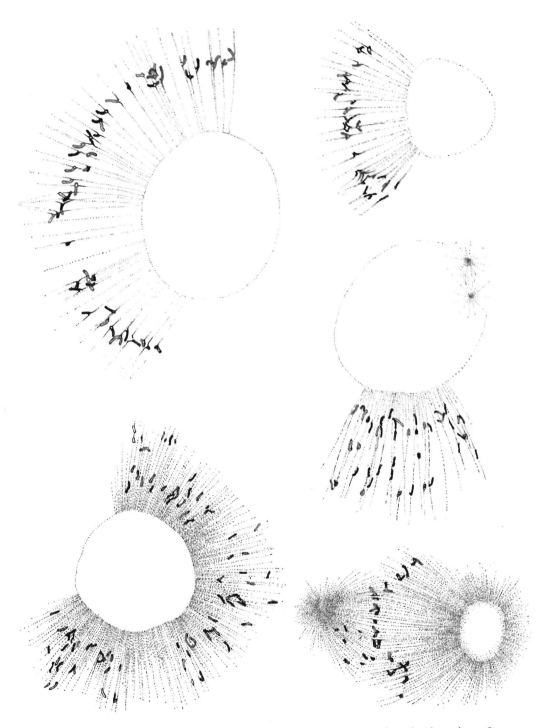

Fig. 11.5 Emil Heitz and Hans Bauer's 1933 illustration of meiosis in the fly, Bibio hortulanus L. Their drawings capture several aspects of the miracle of meiosis by which the chromosomes replicate, come together in pairs around the equator of the cell, recombine (parts of the maternal and paternal chromatids exchange), line up on the spindle, and the two sister chromatids separate from each other and move to opposite poles of the spindle.

twenty cards apart. Genes that are linked tend to stay together in a shuffle, in other words do not segregate independently.

The likelihood with which any two genes stay together is directly proportional to the linear distance between them. The distance is measured in Morgan units in honor of the great biologist, T.H. Morgan, who proved that genes were arrayed on chromosomes. He also discovered four orderly sets of fruit fly genes corresponding to the four pairs of Drosophila chromosomes. If humans could be bred like flies, it would have been possible, thousands of years ago, to infer that we had 23 sets of chromosomes.

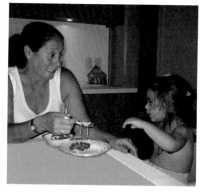

Fig. 11.6 Delicious Brussels sprouts

Linkage and Blood Groups

Decades after evidence that the Kell gene and the gene controlling the ability to taste phenyl thio-carbamide (PTC) were loosely linked, both genes were mapped to the long arm of chromosome 7. A molecule resembling PTC gives members of the cabbage family its bitter taste. About 70% of most populations find PTC bitter and hate Brussels sprouts (Fig. 11.6).

Blood groups have played a significant role in the development of human genetics. Aside from albinism, alkaptonuria and other inborn errors of metabolism, the ABO blood groups were an early example of Mendelian inheritance.

The first example of X-linkage in man was that of hemophilia and color blindness reported by Julia Bell and J.B.S. Haldane in 1937. The first example of autosomal linkage was between Lutheran and the secretor (originally thought to be Lewis) genes by J. Mohr in 1951. Analysis of the *LU:SE* linkage provided the first proof of crossing-over between homologous human chromosomes.

Elliptocytosis was shown to be linked to RH in some families but not in others. This provided the first indication that elliptocytosis, which at the time was considered a single entity, was determined by more than one gene. Today, we know this is indeed true.

Following the initial classification of the autosomes, *FY* became the first gene to be assigned to a specific chromosome through its linkage to an inherited variation in heterochromatin. Furthermore, *XG* was the first nonpathogenic gene to be assigned to the X chromosome. Finally, the first demonstration that sex can influence human chromosomal cross-over frequency came from analyses of linkage data involving blood groups, *LU:SE* and

Mother: "Brussels sprouts are good for you and delicious."
Child: "I can't eat Brussels sprouts because I have PTC taste receptors at the base of my tongue which you, mother dear, lack because you have a mutant allele on the long arm of your number 7 chromosome."

ABO:nail patella syndrome. Xg^a can be used to mark the intricate steps taken as the pairs of chromosomes separate to form sperm and egg. When an X chromosome is gained or lost, as in Klinefelter's or Turner's syndrome, the parental line and the stage at which non-disjunction occurred can be inferred with Xg^a. In addition, X-linked blood group genes provide simple markers to test the Lyon hypothesis.

Inheritance of ABO blood groups

The transferases (enzymes that transfer, or add, a sugar) that are responsible for the expression of the ABO groups are encoded by dominant genes. Group O exists when neither A nor B is present; group O is the result of homozygosity for two recessive genes.

From the nine possible ABO genotypes, some are phenotypically identical (e.g. A/A and A/O); this reduces the possible combinations to six. Further, because of dominance, there are only four phenotypes, A, B, AB and O.

The fact that O is recessive to A and B, means that a child can have a different ABO phenotype from either or both of its parents. Thus, a group A mother and a group B father can have an A, B, AB, or even an O child.

Applications in establishing identity

Starting in the 1930s, inheritance of blood groups was used for settling problems of identity and parentage. The discovery that some twins differed in a single blood group established that they were fraternal twins.

For paternity cases, the detection of a blood group antigen was used to infer the presence of the corresponding gene. To give unequivocal evidence concerning parentage, a characteristic must show Mendelian inheritance, be expressed at birth, and remain unchanged throughout life. Apart from very rare exceptions, where a disease may change an antigen, otherwise they possess all these attributes. Thus, blood groups could resolve forensic and family disputes. Blood groups also were used to determine the identity of babies when doubts arose concerning an accidental switch in a maternity ward. Race and Sanger were involved in an unhappy case in which a young baby had been stolen. The police found a baby but the mother was not sure whether it was hers or not; blood groups showed it was not. The use of blood groups in exclusion of maternity is uncommon. Wiener gives an interesting example. A woman persuaded a man to become her seventh husband saying he was the father of her child. MN groups excluded the woman from being the mother. Subsequently, it was discovered that the child had been obtained from an orphanage.

In 1943, Joan Barry filed a paternity suit against Charlie Chaplin alleging that he had fathered her child. Although blood tests proved Chaplin was not the father, the evidence was not accepted by the unevolved California courts that then ordered him to support the child. Thereafter, California law allowed blood tests as evidence of non paternity. Blood groups can, in the hands of an expert, be used to type blood stains, and ABO groups can be detected from seminal fluid stains, and even saliva on stamps or on cigarette butts!

Blood groups and genetic knowledge

By studying genes encoding the 30 blood group systems, genetic events not found in yeast, fruit flies, or mice were exposed. For example, the three genes comprising the MNS system (*GYPA*, *GYPB*, and *GYPE*), which are homologous and adjacent on chromosome 4, recombine to form hybrid genes. There have been identified "hot spots" where the genes are prone to breaking, thereby allowing recombination if the chromosomes slightly misalign. The recombinations can result in contraction or expansion of the genes. A chromosome with a *GYPA-GYPB* hybrid gene lacks *GYPA* and *GYPB* (contraction) while a chromosome with a *GYPB-GYPA* hybrid gene also possess *GYPA* and *GYPB* (expansion). The hybrid genes were easy to find because they express novel antigens (Fig. 11.7).

RHD and *RHCE* also can form hybrid genes and encode hybrid proteins. These two genes consist of 10 exons (the parts of the gene that encodes a protein). Rather than being in the same orientation on the chromosome, they are juxtaposed (exons 1 to 10 and exons 10 to 1). As an unrelated gene resides between *RHD* and *RHCE*, there is enough room for a hairpin bend so the two genes align and the exchange of nucleotides from *RHD* to *RHCE*, or from *RHCE* to *RHD*, is not uncommon (Fig. 11.8).

The *GYPC* revealed that two products can be encoded by the same gene. This gene has two "start" codons (AUG). If the first one is used, glycophorin C (GPC) is encoded; if the second one is

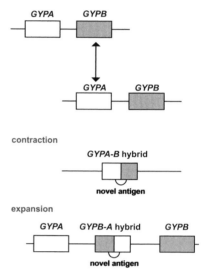

Fig. 11.7 Cross-over between *GYPA* and *GYPB* on misaligned chromosomes results in a contraction and expansion

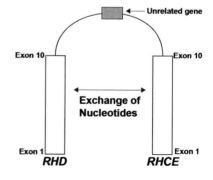

Fig. 11.8 Transfer of nucleotide between *RHD* and *RHCE*

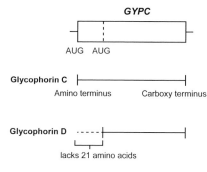

Fig. 11.9 Two protein products from one gene

used, glycophorin D (GPD) is encoded. GPD is a truncated version of GPC lacking 21 amino acid residues from its amino terminus (Fig. 11.9).

Just as investigations of blood groups have shed light on the field of human genetics, the reverse is now the case. Testing of DNA is now used to predict the presence or absence of a blood group. Technical advances in genetics and molecular biology have provided blood group scientists with the opportunity to further their discipline. As a result, information regarding the chromosome location, DNA sequence, nucleotide variation, and regulatory elements of genes controlling expression of blood groups has been elucidated. The relationship between blood groups and disease were for a long time only statistical associations, but they can now be established or rejected through the power of biochemistry, bacteriology, and immunology.

Chapter 12   Power of Techniques

> Progress in science depends on new techniques, new dis-
> coveries and new ideas, probably in that order.
>
> —Sydney Brenner

Just as the discovery of America was dependent on the sailing ship, the compass, and the confidence that one was not going to fall off the edge, the discovery and elucidation of blood group antigens was dependent on an array of technologies, and the concept that antigens were encoded by physical genes, whose sequence can be laid bare even from a pinprick of blood. As technology advanced, so did our comprehension of the role played by blood groups—or, more precisely, by the membrane component on which they are carried.

The first few blood group antibody/antigen interactions were detected by the direct agglutination test, which was possible because the antigens are abundant. However, the majority were found by the antiglobulin test, which is the primary test for detecting IgG antibodies. Although the antiglobulin test was discovered at the end of World War II, amazingly it has not been superseded by a better test to detect antibody/antigen interactions.

As carbohydrate biochemical techniques were applied to the study of blood groups, the specific carbohydrates detected by direct agglutinating antibodies were revealed. These studies showed that the terminal sugar of the A antigen is N-acetylgalactosamine, for B it is galactose, and for H it is fucose. The difference between A and B sugars is readily recognized by the immune system. The antibodies (anti-A and anti-B) are IgM and IgG and are important in terms of blood transfusion. The ability of the immune system to recognize the very small differences in these sugars illustrates that old fashioned direct agglutination is a wonderful technique.

In the 1970s and 1980s, sodium dodecyl sulphate (SDS)-poly-acylamide gel electrophoresis (PAGE) was used to separate and identify proteins that make up the red cell membrane. SDS-PAGE, together with western[1] blotting (the transfer of proteins from the gel to a paper-like support medium that can be probed with antibody) further enhanced the study of many red cell membrane glycoproteins.

These studies have led to the unraveling of major constituents of the red cell membrane, which can be likened to a piece of embroidery. The material is equivalent to the lipid bilayer and its underlying skeleton, while the colorful threads in a variety of stitches are equivalent to the variety of proteins and glycoproteins in the red cell membrane. The blood groups are like shells or beads sewn onto the embroidered pictures. Blood groups made a major contribution to the development of the knowledge regarding the components of membranes.

When it was possible to make monoclonal antibodies that detected blood group antigens, our ability to consistently detect antigens, by both agglutination and western blotting, changed dramatically. As monoclonal antibodies generally agglutinate red cells more strongly than their polyclonal counterparts, antigens carried on proteins with low copy number per red cell can be detected reliably. For example, monoclonal antibodies readily detect, in the direct agglutination test, some weak forms of the D antigen. The term D[u] is now obsolete. D[u] was used to define D antigens that were not detected by polyclonal antibodies by direct agglutination testing but were detected by the indirect antiglobulin test—the "u" came from undeveloped.

The ability to clone and sequence nucleotides provided insights into genes encoding blood group systems. The revolutionary polymerase chain reaction (PCR), led to the ability to amplify a piece of DNA to predict the presence or absence of a blood group antigen or even to blood type a mammoth or an Egyptian mummy. With the invention of the PCR machine, this methodology became widely available. This technique can be applied to high throughput DNA array platforms, thereby providing the potential to screen a large number of blood donors to increase inventories of antigen-negative blood components for transfusion.

Another key use of PCR is to predict the phenotype of a recently transfused patient because donor red cells in the recipient's circulation do not interfere with the test. A further key use is to predict the antigen type of a fetus at risk for HDN. When a pregnant woman has an IgG antibody that could pass through the placenta, knowing the blood type of the fetus is of immense value. If the

1. The British biologist Edwin Southern first detected DNA sequences with hybridizing probes on DNA fragments separated electrophoretically. Variant methods relying on the same principle were playfully called northern blots for analyzing RNA and western blots for analyzing proteins.

fetus is predicted to lack the antigen corresponding to the mother's antibody, then the mother need not be monitored or endure invasive procedures during her pregnancy. Fetal DNA can be obtained from amniocytes or maternal plasma. Prediction of the blood type of the fetus is particularly valuable when a mother's plasma contains anti-K, anti-Kp^a, or anti-Ge3 because the titer does not predict whether the fetus is antigen-positive or the severity of HDN. These antibodies, in addition to causing immune destruction, also suppress erythropoiesis. This can result in a severely anemic and hydropic neonate. The Kell protein and glycophorin C (protein expressing antigens in the Ge system) are expressed on very early erythroid progenitor cells (BFU-E and CFU-E). It has been shown in vitro that anti-K and anti-Ge3 suppress the growth of erythroid progenitor cells. In the case of anti-Ge3, the antibody may inhibit a protein kinase through which erythropoietin achieves its effects.

As techniques changed and became commonplace, and as typed red cells and characterized antibodies (in human plasma, lectins, monoclonals) became available, antibody identification and antigen determinations were performed in many laboratories worldwide. The number of investigators who made a contribution is too large to give all their due.

In addition to the well-established importance of blood groups to transfusion and transplantation medicine, their study has had a significant effect on human genetics and other branches of biology. Some of the contributions, especially associations of blood groups to disease, will be discussed in the next chapter.

| Chapter 13 | **Blood Groups and Disease** |

On Monday when the sun is hot
I wonder to myself a lot:
Now is it true or is it not
That what is which and which is what.

—A.A. Milne

Reports of far-fetched links between blood groups and disease have been claimed, many based on statistical analyses. Early studies were often controversial because the number of people studied was small, controls were inadequate, or data were incorrectly analyzed. Even when all these caveats have been avoided, statistical associations alone are insufficient to indicate cause. In R.A. Fisher's booklet casting doubt on smoking as a cause of cancer, he cited the strong correlation between the increase in divorce and the increase in the importation of green apples in England as an example of statistical associations not necessarily being causal. Nevertheless, from the collective body of statistical data, there emerged associations between blood groups and bleeding disorders, malignancy, and infection. Some of these statistical relationships appeared to have no logical connection but they have been verified experimentally.

R.A. Fisher proposed that R. Doll and A.B. Hill's finding of an association between cigarette smoking and cancer might equally well be explained by incipient cancer provoking smoking or perhaps some other factor, such as a gene that might cause both. This was hard to believe unless you were a paid adviser to the tobacco industry, which Fisher was. Similarly, Wiener always maintained that LW and Rh were the same antigen. This was hard to believe unless your being the discoverer of Rh depended on it.

Improbable associations

Examples of hard-to-believe associations include claims that group A people have the worst hangovers, group B people defecate most and are predisposed to crime, group B females have more off-spring, and group O people have the best teeth! Blood groups have been proposed to indicate personality traits. In 1973, a paper was published in *Nature* on a relationship between ABO groups and intelligence: group A_2 people were said to have the highest IQ, and group A_1 people the lowest IQ, and group O people fell in between. In 1983, the same journal published a paper making the claim that, in the British population, group A is significantly more common among members of the higher socioeconomic groups. The paper was entitled: "ABO genes are differentially distributed in socio-economic groups in England." Plausibility or the lack thereof no less than papers in learned journals have not been per-fect predictors of truth; Darwin said: "I have no faith in anything short of actual measurement and the rule of three."

Large companies in Japan specify the desired blood group when advertising for, and evaluating, job applicants. Group A people are thought to be more detail oriented and best suited for jobs requiring accuracy. A book on the 1998 *New York Times* best seller list, *Eat Right 4 Your Type*, suggests there is a strong asso-ciation between blood groups and digestion and that one should formulate a diet according to one's blood group. A second book by the same author provided special diets for each of the four ABO groups. The basic premise presented in the first book is that group O was the original blood group and that people of this type were hunter-gatherers and meat eaters. In contrast, it is claimed, later generations who were group A became farmers and ate more grains and vegetables, and drank milk. Groups B and AB were said to be the last to emerge because of racial intermingling. It turns out that this assertion is completely wrong. Results of studies on DNA from the ABO blood group alleles show that the O gene is a variant of the A gene. Thus, group O actually appeared later than the other ABO groups!

Could epidemics explain the different proportions of ABO groups in different populations? It is possible that certain epidem-ics were responsible. For instance, some differences may be a con-sequence of an "A-like" antigen on the smallpox virus, and an "H-like" antigen on the plague bacillus and on *Vibrio cholerae*. These look-alike antigens could render individuals who have an-ti-A (groups B and O) more resistant to smallpox, and individuals who can make anti-H (groups AB, A_1, and B) more resistant to the plague and cholera.

The prehuman species, *hominoid*, diverged from chimpanzees

Table 13.1 Some associations of blood groups with infections

Infection	Blood Group with a Higher Incidence of Disease
Plague	O
Cholera	O
Mumps	O
Helicobacter pylori	O
Leprosy: Tuberculoid form	O
Lepromatous form	A, B
Tuberculosis	O, B
Giardia lamblia	A
Smallpox	A, AB
Gonorrhea	B
Streptococcus pneumoniae	B
Escherichia coli	B, AB
Salmonella	B, AB
Neisseria meningitidis	Non-secretor of ABH
Haemophilus influenzae	Non-secretor of ABH
Candida albicans	Non-secretor of ABH
Malaria	Duffy glycophorine A

6 to 8 million years ago. The hominoid group O variant began to emerge 5 million years ago, before *Homo sapiens* began to emerge in Africa approximately 200,000 years ago. It is postulated that during the years from the origin of *Homo sapiens* to their migration out of Africa, there might have been a gradual increase in the prevalence of group O because there is evidence that O confers resistance to severe *Plasmodium falciparum* infection.

Associations of blood groups with alkaline phosphatase and coagulation factors

Using starch-gel electrophoresis, human plasma alkaline phosphatase can be separated into a fast-moving and a slow-moving component. The fast-moving component is present in plasma from all ABO groups, whereas the slow-moving component is present in easily detectable levels in plasma of group B and O secretors, in small amounts in 10% to 15% of group A secretors, and in trace amounts in non-secretors of any group. Alkaline phosphatases are present in many human tissues, including bone, intestine, kidney, liver, placenta, and leukocytes where they may function as part of a membrane pump for calcium and phosphorus. Ingestion of fat stimulates the appearance of alkaline phosphatase. Factors involved in the amount of alkaline phosphate may influence fat handling in the intestine.

There is a statistical association suggesting that group O and A_2 occur less frequently in people with venous thromboembolism. This may be because they have lower levels of factors VIII (antihemophilic globulin), V, IX, and von Willebrand factor.

Associations of blood groups and malignancy

Group A dominates over group O in many cancers of the digestive system, and of the uterus and cervix. The relative increase of group A to O is 1.64 in salivary gland cancer; 1.28 in cancer of the ovaries, and 1.22 in stomach cancer. Although these associations were initially based on statistical analyses, there is now additional evidence to support the claims.

As cells become malignant, they tend to lose their original antigens and acquire new ones, called tumor antigens. These "new" antigens are sometimes precursors of antigens normally present, or are "illegitimate" antigens, that is, antigens not under genetic control by the host. The number of ABO antigens can diminish on malignant cells as the malignancy progresses, and their loss is proportional to the metastatic potential of the tumor. Some tumor antigens have properties similar to the A antigen ("A-like") that cross-react with anti-A. If tumor "A-like"antigens are recognized by the host's immune system as foreign, group O or group B patients (who do have anti-A) would be less susceptible to tumor growth compared to group A patients (who do not have anti-A).

An antibody called anti-PP1P^k (originally anti-Tj^a, now renamed anti-GLOB), was found in plasma from a patient named Mrs. Jay with a gastric adenocarcinoma. An extract of the tumor inhibited the activity of the antibody, hence the name "T"for tumor, "j" for Jay. The patient, who was later shown to be the first person with the p phenotype (PP1P^k–, P$_{null}$) was given a small volume of incompatible blood, which resulted in a severe hemolytic transfusion reaction and boosted the strength of the antibody. After a subtotal gastrectomy, she survived for 22 years without any evidence of tumor recurrence or metastasis. In contrast, her sister, who also was of the same rare phenotype and not given incompatible blood, died of adenocarcinoma of the uterus. Levine suggested adenocarcinomas in these p patients had produced an "illegitimate" P antigen, and Mrs. Jay's hyper-immune response to the incompatible blood had led to the destruction of malignant cells expressing P antigen. In 1982, the major glycolipid isolated from Mrs. Jay's tumor, which had been stored, was shown to have "illegitimate" P specificity. Remarkable but true!

P is part of globoside, which is a chain of specific carbohydrates attached to a lipid (Fig. 14.1). Globoside is the receptor of human parvovirus B19, the virus that causes fifth disease (so-called because it then was the 5th most common disease of childhood). This virus and some strains of E. coli use the disaccharide, galactose-galactose, present in P1, P, and P^k antigens on epithelial cells lining the urethra to gain entry to the urinary tract. People with the p phenotype are found among the Amish and Finns, and very rarely among others: they lack this disaccharide and are immune to parvovirus B19 and E. coli.

Another connection between blood groups and malignancies occurs when terminal sugars are released, exposing a sugar that was previously hidden. One example is the Forssman[1] antigen that is structurally similar to the A antigen. Most human plasma samples contain naturally occurring anti-Forssman antibodies that

1. In 1911, John F. Forssman showed that a variety of antigens could stimulate an antibody (called anti-Forssman, in his honor) in humans that lysed sheep red cells. These were called heterophile antigens, because they occurred in different species and had a similar structure. Although the antigens are not identical, the immune response is indistinguishable. Anti-Forssman is commonly found in people with infectious mononucleosis.

Bacteriology became a defined discipline in Lund in 1888 and Forssman was the first professor of the subject, overseeing research into botulism and staphylococcal toxins; among others. Venereal disease was a big problem in the 19th century and a special "Cure House" was built in Lund. As Professor of General Health Care in the early 1900s, Forssman was in charge of this clinic that was nicknamed "The Sailors' Home in Lund."

agglutinate or lyse red cells expressing Forssman antigen (e.g. sheep red cells). Anti-Forssman cross-reacts with A and P antigens on human red cells. While Forssman antigen is not detected in normal gastrointestinal mucosa, gastric tumors express Forssman antigen.

The "illegitimate" Forssman antigen in malignant tissue may account for up to 15% of the "A-like" antigens. Other "illegitimate" A antigens include Tn antigens. T and Tn antigens are not present on normal breast tissue but can be expressed by breast cancers and other malignancies. Delayed hypersensitivity tests, where T and Tn antigens were injected intradermally, showed no reactions in normal subjects, a small number of positive reactions in patients with benign tumors, and a high number of positive reactions in patients with cancer. This suggests T and Tn blood group antigens are involved in a cellular immune response in cancer.

Presence of Tn antigen on red cells results in a form of polyagglutination (red cells expressing Tn or T are agglutinated by plasma from most adults) but Tn differs from T in that the Tn antigen is persistently, not transiently, uncovered. Expression of Tn is caused by a somatic mutation of the gene encoding galactosyl transferase. As the mutation occurs in some, not all, stem cells, a proportion of the normal O-glycans (a chain of four sugars attached to serine or threonine) are incompletely formed, leaving exposed an N-acetylgalactosamine sugar (Fig. 13.1). There is a mixture of normally glycosylated red cells and Tn-active aberrantly glycosylated red cells, which leads to the classic mixed-field appearance of this type of polyagglutination.

Tn, discovered 30 years after T, took its name from Tannenbaum, the first proband with Tn, who had an undefined hemolytic condition. Tn polyagglutination is associated with myelodysplastic syndrome, a condition that may progress to leukemia.

Associations with peptic ulcers

In the mid 1950s, statistical associations between peptic ulcers and ABO groups were noted. Group O people are 20% more likely than group A people to have peptic ulcers. Duodenal ulcers were 35% more likely to develop in group O people compared with group A, B, and AB people, and 50% more likely to develop in people who are non-secretors. Non-secretors of ABH account for 20% of the population. Putting these numbers together, group O non-secretors are 2½ times more likely to have a duodenal ulcer

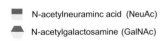

■ N-acetylneuraminc acid (NeuAc)

▲ N-acetylgalactosamine (GalNAc)

Somatic Mutation

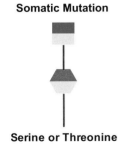

Serine or Threonine

Fig. 13.1 Tn antigen results from a lack of one galactose and one neuraminic acid molecule

than group A, B, or AB secretors.

In 1982, Barry Marshall and Robin Warren discovered a new species of bacterium, *Helicobacter pylori,* living in the stomach where it sometimes caused inflammation, ulceration and cancer. In 1993, the Lewis blood group antigen, Le^b (which has close associations with the ABO system), was shown to be the receptor for *Helicobacter pylori*. As group A people have fewer Le^b antigens, there are fewer sites for the bacteria to attach. This provides a rationale for the observation that gastric ulcers are much more common in group O than in group A people.

Associations with infections

As described in Chapter 2, Springer and colleagues showed that many bacteria (e.g. *Escherichia coli)* have molecules on their membranes that resemble A or B blood group antigens. Expression of these look-alike antigens on microorganisms is the stimulus for anti-A and anti-B production by humans. Other antibodies that occur in plasma without apparent immunization (e.g. anti-I, anti-T, anti-Tk, anti-Tn) are also thought to be antibodies to bacteria that cross-react with red cells.

Clear cut connections between blood groups and infections involve enzymes that are produced by the bacteria. The enzymes cleave sugars from the surface of the red cell exposing hidden antigens such that they are agglutinated by plasma from most humans. Some microorganisms (e.g. *Vibrio cholerae, Clostridia perfringens,* pneumococci, influenza virus) produce neuraminidase. This pugnacious enzyme releases sialic acid from sugar chains attached to proteins in the red cell membrane (mainly the glycophorins) and uncovers carbohydrates (galactose linked to N-acetyl-galactosamine) (Figure 13.2). This disaccharide is called the T antigen, named by Friendenreich to honor his teacher, Thomsen, who first reported this cryptantigen in 1927 that he named "L". Activation of the T antigen is associated with septicemia.

Other microorganisms (*Bacteroides fragilis, Aspergillus niger, Serratia marcescens, Candida albicans*) produce a different enzyme, called galacosidase that cleaves galactose from N-acetyl-glucosamine in complex carbohydrate structures. This action exposes the Tk antigen, (Fig. 13.3), which was named "T", because of its similarity to T polyagglutination and "k" from the proband H.K. A third form of related polyagglutination, Th, was named after the

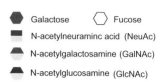

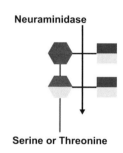

Fig. 13.2 T antigen revealed after cleavage of two neuraminic acid molecules

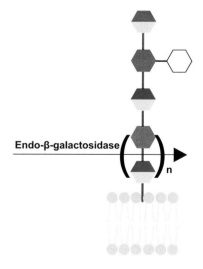

Fig. 13.3 Tk antigen revealed after cleavage of galactose and N-acetylglucosamine molecules

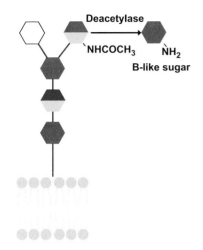

Deacetylase

NHCOCH₃   NH₂

B-like sugar

Fig. 13.4 Acquired B like antigen results when the NHCOCH3 side arm on the A sugar (GalNAc) is converted to a NH2 side arm, which is similar to the B sugar

proband, Anne Harbidge. The association between exposure of Tk and Th antigens and infections by one of these organisms, if they cause septicemia, is clear.

Another enzyme, produced by the bacterium *Escherichia coli* called deacetylase, alters the $NHCOCH_3$ side chain on N-acetyl galactosamine (the A blood group) to a NH_2 side chain (Fig. 13.4). This altered sugar resembles blood group B and is agglutinated by anti-B. This altered sugar is called "acquired B" and its presence is associated with colon cancer. The tumor causes lesions in the colon wall allowing *E. coli* to migrate into the blood stream.

People with the rare congenital disorder called leukocyte adhesion deficiency syndrome (LAD II or congenital disorder of glycosylation II), who are mostly from the Middle East, suffer recurrent bacterial infections. Red cells from these patients lack all antigens in ABO and Lewis blood group systems (Bombay phenotype). The underlying cause is a mutation in the gene that encodes the fucose transporter. Without this protein, fucose cannot be transported into cells, which is a prerequisite for expression of H (the H antigen is fucose, the precursor to A, B, and Le antigens), A, B, and sLe^X. Without sLe^X, neutrophils cannot roll and ingest bacteria. The patients are treated temporarily with high doses of oral fucose or permanently with bone marrow transplant. Red cells that lack A, B, and H antigens are said to have the "Bombay" phenotype (albeit caused by a different mechanism) because the first few probands were from Bombay—before it was renamed Mumbai. Although the defect is not primarily one of the red cell, typing red cells for A, B, H, Le^a, and Le^b is a simple way to diagnose LAD II in patients with high white blood cell counts and chronic infections.

An absence of the Xk protein (Kx_{null}, McLeod phenotype) can be caused by a deletion of part of the X chromosome that encompasses the *XK* gene and a neighboring gene, *Phox-91*. Lack of *XK* gives rise to the McLeod syndrome and lack of *Phox-91* gives rise to X-linked chronic granulomatous disease (CGD). CGD is usually discovered in children and manifests as recurrent life-threatening bacterial and fungal infections. The disease is caused by ineffective phagocytosis.

Other Disease Associations

Tables 13.2 and 13.3 summarize some other diseases associated with blood group antigens.

Table 13.2 Summary of infections and diseases and associated alteration of antigen expression

Condition	Antigens affected
AIDS	Knops
AIHA	Enᵃ, U, Rh, Kell, Jkᵃ, LW, Gerbich, Scianna, Vel, Diego, AnWj
Alcoholic cirrhosis	Lewis
Carcinoma	A, B, H, I, P1, Knops
Diseases with increased clearance of immune complexes	Knops
Increased hemopoiesis	A, B, H, I (concomitant increased expression of i)
Hodgkin's disease	A, B, H, LW, Colton
Infection	A, B, H, I, A with appearance of Tn, A with appearance of acquired B, K
Infectious mononucleosis	Lewis
LADII	A, B, H, Lewis
Leukemia	A, B, H, I, Rh, Ytᵃ, Colton
Old age	JMH, A, B, H
PNH	Cromer, Yt, Dombrock, MER2
Pregnancy	A, B, H, I, Lewis, LW, P1, JMH, Sdᵃ, some Jkᵃ, Gyᵃ and AnWj
SE Asian ovalocytosis	Enᵃ, S, s, U, Diᵇ, Wrᵇ, D, C, e, Kpᵇ, Jkᵃ, Jkᵇ, Xgᵃ, LW, Sc1
SLE	Chido/Rodgers; Knops; Ytᵃ
Splenic infarctions, inflammatory bowel disease	Cromer
Thalassemia	I

Table 13.3 Blood groups associated with disease susceptibility

Blood Group	Disease Susceptibility
Group A	Carcinoma of the salivary glands, stomach, colon, rectum, ovary, uterus, cervix, bladder; idiopathic thrombocytopenic purpura, coronary thrombosis, thrombosis (oral contraceptives), pernicious anemia, giardiasis, meningococcal meningitis
Group B	*Escherichia coli* urinary tract infection, gonorrhea
Group O	Duodenal and gastric ulcers, rheumatoid arthritis, von Willebrand disease, typhoid, paratyphoid, cholera
ABH nonsecretors	Duodenal ulcer, spondyloarthropathy; increased susceptibility to *Candida albicans*, *Neisseria meningitis*, *Streptococcus pneumonia*, *Haemophilus influenzae*
Le(a–b–)	Sjögren's syndrome
Group O, Le(a–b+)	Peptic ulceration (*Helicobacter pylori*)
Globoside	Fifth disease (Parvovirus)

Racial associations

Some blood groups differ among different populations. Fig. 13.5 shows the percentages of ABO, D, K, Fy^a, Fy^b, Jk^a, and Jk^b phenotypes in Asians, African Americans and Caucasians. These differences are significant in transfusion medicine. If a patient requires blood lacking, say, K, Fy^a, and Jk^b antigens, it would be necessary to test only two African Americans to find one suitable donor, but 10 Caucasians, and 100 Asians. For the majority of patients who do not have the antibodies, selection of antigen-negative blood is unnecessary and one can ignore these ethnic differences. Interestingly, 100% of the Parakanã tribe of South American Indians from the Para region of the Amazon have group O blood type.

Table 13.4 gives examples of blood groups and the ethnicity where each is most likely to be found. The blood groups listed are rare, but the knowledge is useful. Obviously, it is more fruitful to search for a blood group where it is known to exist, thus racial profiling has its place, particularly to help the ethnic group being profiled. This is a far cry from prejudices that arose about the quality of blood between races. Until the middle of the 20th century, blood from African Americans was considered different from, and inferior to, blood from Caucasians, just as the brains of women were considered to be different from, and inferior to, the brains of men.

While most seemingly absurd associations are absurd there have been many other associations between blood group antigens and disease that have been transformed into respectable established facts—surprising many. As appropriate techniques became available, other associations have been revealed and will be disclosed in the next chapter.

Table 13.4 Antigens and ethnic associations

Blood group antigens	Ethnic group
Kp(a+b–)	Caucasian
Js(a+b–)	African
Jk(a–b–)	Polynesian
Ok(a–)	Japanese
Ge:–2,–3	Papua New Guinean
Yt(a–b+)	Arabs, Israeli
SERF–	Thais
In(a+b–)	Indian
GUTI–	Chilean
Di(a+b–)	East Asians, Native Americans
Fr(a+)	Mennonites
DANE+	Danes
Evans+	Celts
He+	Xhosas
Hil+	Chinese
KREP+	Poles
Mg+	Swiss
Vr+	Dutch
Wb+	Welsh
Wd(a+)	Hutterites

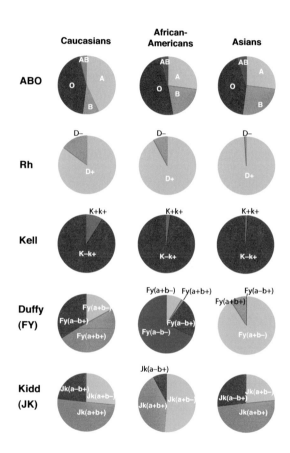

Fig. 13.5 Pie chart showing racial distribution of some blood types

Chapter 14   **Blood Groups and Immunity**

Curiouser and curiouser!

—Lewis Carroll

As statistical associations gave way to proof of the causal connections between blood groups and diseases, the associations became in some ways even more curious. This chapter reviews some links between antibody production and membrane proteins and diseases associated with them. It is not the blood group antigens themselves that are important, but the membrane component. Indeed, the amino acid changes that give rise to expression of the actual blood group antigens are almost invariably in non-critical parts of the protein. However, their absence from membrane proteins with immunologically important functions has led to antibody production that revealed aspects of biological importance.

Antibodies

Antibodies to many blood group antigens are not just associated with, but are the cause of, hemolytic transfusion reactions and hemolytic disease of the newborn. The percentage of people whose plasma contains acquired antibodies varies. An average figure for blood donors is 0.2%, but for women who have been pregnant it is 0.4%, for transfused patients 0.6%, and for patients with sickle cell disease the figure can be as high as 35%. Anti-K is the now the commonest antibody, anti-D is the second most common, followed by antibodies to E, c, e, C, Fy^a, Fy^b, Jk^a, Jk^b, and S antigens.

Antibodies to blood groups also cause autoimmune hemolytic anemia (AIHA)—both the cold type and the warm type. Autoimmune hemolytic anemia is a collective term used when a person's immune system makes antibodies to antigens on their own red cells. Such antibodies lead to the premature removal of red cells from the patient's circulation, and thus, anemia. AIHA can occur as a side effect of drugs or some diseases.

In some healthy people, antibodies are sometimes produced against a normal component of the red cell membrane without apparent cause and, once started, exposure to cold can provoke hemolysis. The antibodies can cause anemia, rejection of a graft, spontaneous abortion and other diseases. Three interesting correlations between antibodies to blood group antigens are now summarized.

First, women with certain quite rare antibodies, namely anti-PP1P^k and anti-P, have a higher than normal rate of spontaneous abortions in the first trimester. A person with p phenotype can make anti-PP1P^k, a person with the P^k phenotype can make anti-P. These antibodies tend to cause hemolysis causing many to abort. Plasmapheresis has been used to reduce the amount of antibody in the plasma of women with the p or P^k phenotype. As a consequence they have delivered viable infants. The use of plasmapheresis for this purpose was pioneered at Johns Hopkins Hospital in Baltimore. Cyril Levene, Director of the Blood Group Reference Laboratory in Jerusalem, tells an interesting anecdote, relating to a patient with the p phenotype.

> During the investigation of a family of a woman who was p, we found that two of her siblings were also p. One was a brother, and the other her sister. This sister was group O and had a history of spontaneous abortions and no live child. The religious law in Israel states that if a woman is incapable of childbirth, it is grounds for divorce!

One night in late 1984, she heard on the radio about this new procedure that had been carried out at Johns Hopkins Hospital, in Baltimore. Dr Levene contacted Dr Paul Ness, Director of the Transfusion Service at Johns Hopkins Hospital, who sent over their plasmapheresis protocol. The plasmapheresis was duly performed in the Rambam Hospital in Haifa and the woman eventually delivered a live child. "We wrote to Dr Ness and told him that in Hebrew 'Ness' means 'Miracle' and indeed plasmapheresis was for this patient of ours."

The second is paroxysmal cold hemoglobinuria (PCH), (a rare type of cold AIHA) in which an autoantibody (anti-P), when bound to the patient's red cells, binds complement and causes

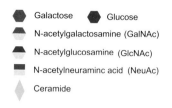

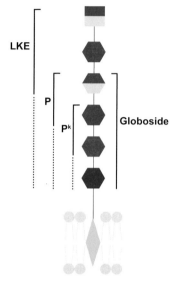

Fig. 14.1 Carbohydrates associated with expression of P and P^k antigen

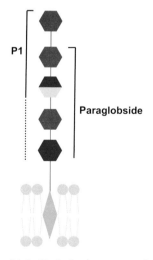

Fig. 14.2 Carbohydrates associated with expression of P1 antigen

1. Julius Donath and Karl Landsteiner investigated paroxysmal cold hemoglobinuria in 1904. They discovered that it was due to an autoantibody, something that Ehrlich had stated could not exist. It was later shown to be an IgG antibody usually against the P antigen. In addition to describing the first autoimmune disease, they demonstrated in the laboratory that cooling a blood sample from a patient to 4°C would attach a heat sensitive antibody to the red cells, and would hemolyse when warmed, due to activation of the complement cascade. Donath studied in Vienna, graduating as an MD in 1895, the same year as Landsteiner.

hemolysis after the patient is exposed to cold temperatures. This autoantibody is called the Donath-Landsteiner[1] (D-L) antibody after Donath and Landsteiner who developed the diagnostic test that is still in use today. PCH is characterized by sudden severe hemolysis, causing hemoglobinuria. Typically, PCH follows an infection that triggers production of antibodies that cross-react with the P antigen on the red cell membrane. PCH can be caused by the body's response to viral infections such as measles, mumps, influenza, adenovirus, chickenpox, cytomegalovirus, and Epstein-Barr virus, and to bacterial infections such as syphilis, *Haemophilus influenzae* and *Mycoplasma pneumoniae*. Patients with PCH should avoid the cold; even air conditioning can trigger hemolysis.

Table 14-1 Diseases associated with antibody production

Antibody specificity	Associated diseases/conditions
Most IgG	Transfusion reactions
Most IgG	Hemolytic disease of the newborn
Anti-I, -IH, -i, -H, -Pr	Cold agglutinin disease
Anti-"Rh," -"Kell," -U, -Wr^b	Warm autoimmune hemolytic anemia
Anti-I	*Mycoplasma pneumoniae*, chronic lymphocytic leukemia, Hodgkin's disease and non-Hodgkin's lymphomas
Anti-i	Infectious mononucleosis, reticuloendothelial diseases
Anti-I^T	Hodgkin's disease and non-Hodgkin's lymphomas
Anti-K	Enterocolitis, bacterial infections (*E. coli* 0125:B15, *Campylobacter jejuni, E. coli*)
Anti-P1	Parasite infections: hydatid cysts, liver flukes
Anti-PP1P^k	Early spontaneous abortions
Anti-P	Paroxysmal cold hemoglobinuria, early spontaneous abortions, lymphoma
Anti-Nf	Renal dialysis
Anti-Forssman	Neoplastic disorders
Anti-Rx	Virally induced hemolysis
Decreased anti-A or B	Agammaglobulinemia or hypogammaglobulinemia

The third association is an antibody in the plasma from patients treated with dialysis for kidney disease. The antibody agglutinated N+ but not N– red cells. The culprit turned out to be the formaldehyde that was used to sterilize the dialysis machines between patients. Trace amounts of formaldehyde entered the patient's circulation and modified the N antigen. The modification was recognized by the patient's immune system as being foreign and produced an antibody that reacted like anti-N. To differentiate it from "normal" anti-N, this antibody was named anti-Nf or anti-Nform. Anti-Nf has an affinity for N on red cells that have been exposed to formaldehyde that is 100 –200 times greater than its affinity to N on untreated red cells. In the United States, this antibody is no longer found because dialysis machines are sterilized with heat or gas and once used, supplies are thrown away.

Antibodies to blood group antigens are made by a small proportion of patients with certain infections, for example Mycoplasma pneumoniae, infectious mononucleosis, and *E. coli* colitis, and have also been made in response to certain malignancies, e.g. Hodgkin's disease and non-Hodgkin's lymphoma (See Table 14.1).

Altered antigen expression in vivo

In certain diseases, antigens on red cells are occasionally altered. They can be enhanced or weakened, or even acquired (Table 14.2).

Increased erythropoiesis can lead to an altered expression of blood groups. Insufficient processing time in the Golgi apparatus has at least two outcomes: (a) there is time for the addition of the first few sugar residues in a carbohydrate chain but not for the terminal sugars. Thus, expression of A or B antigens is weakened. (b) There is less time for carbohydrate chains to form branches. Thus, the I antigen (dependant on branched chains) is expressed more weakly and its reciprocal antigen, i, (expressed on linear carbohydrate chains) is expressed more strongly. In addition, reticulocytes have a weakened expression of some blood group antigens.

The weakened expression of A and B antigens occurs in association with exposure of T, Tk, Th, and Tn antigens. In patients with acute leukemia and aplastic anemia, expression of A and B antigens on red cells can decrease to the extent that they are not detectable by routine methods. The disease induces defects in gly-

Table 14.2 Diseases associated with altered antigen expression

Affected antigen	Disease
Enhanced i and weakened I	Thalassemia, sickle cell disease, HEMPAS, Diamond-Blackfan anemia, myeloblastic or sideroblastic erythropoiesis, refractory anemia, HEMPAS*
Weakened A and/or B	Leukemia, myelodysplastic syndrome, Hodgkin's disease and non-Hodgkin's lymphomas, aplastic anemia, bacterial infections
Weakened MN	Bacterial infections, myelodysplastic syndrome, leukemia (Tn, T, Tk activation)
Weakened target antigens (e.g., Rh, Kell, Kidd, LW)	Autoimmune hemolytic anemia
Weakened I, Rh, S, s, U, Kp^b, Jk^a, Xg^a, or En^a	Stomatocytic hereditary elliptocytosis
Acquired A (Tn)	Myelodysplastic syndrome, acute myelogenous leukemia
Acquired B	Bacterial infections, gastrointestinal ulcers or malignancies
Acquired T, Tk, Th	Bacterial infections
Acquired K antigens	*Enterococcus faecium* infections
Acquired Jk^b antigen	*E. faecium* or *Micrococcus* infection

*a congenital anemia; HEMPAS = hereditary erythroblastic multinuclearity with positive acidified serum lysis test (quite a name for a disease!)

cosyl transferases that are responsible for adding A or B sugars to a carbohydrate chain. As the patient recovers, the antigen expression returns to its former state.

There are also reports of temporary suppression of blood group antigens and formation of an apparent alloantibody. Apparent, at the time, because it does not react with the patient's red cells, but will react after the antigens reappear on the patient's red cells. At this time the antibody is usually not demonstrable in the patient's plasma; thus, the tests have to be done with stored patient sera. These autoantibodies are known as 'mimicking' antibodies—because the autoantibody mimics an alloantibody. The reason for antigen suppression is unknown and uncommon, but the phenomenon occurs in patients with a wide range of diagnoses. There are reports of red cells acquiring K and Jk^b antigens; both thought to be due to adsorption of bacterial antigens.

In AIHA, the autoantibody reacts with a component on the patient's red cells. Sometimes the antibody is specific for a blood group antigen. In AIHA, when the autoantibody reacts with a blood group antigen, it may weaken or ablate its expression.

During pregnancy, Le^a and Le^b antigens are often weakened, as are LW and In^b antigens. Males with the rare McLeod syndrome have a weak expression of antigens in the Kell blood group system.

Altered antigen expression in vitro

Red cells stored in EDTA have a weakened expression of LW antigens. This is because the antigen expression requires magnesium ions, which are chelated by EDTA. Kell antigens are weakened or destroyed if they come into contact with acid or sulfydryl compounds. Due to sulfide bonds, the Kell protein is highly folded. Incubating red cells in sulfydryl compounds breaks these bonds and uncurls the Kell glycoprotein, which alters its conformation and weakens or destroys expression of Kell antigens.

Immunologically important proteins

Several proteins that carry blood group antigens have a biological role, but this role is related to the presence of the protein on other cells in the body and not to the blood group per se. Some of these proteins have immunologically important functions (Table 14.3).

Cell adhesion molecules (CAMs) are immunologically important and participate in cell-to-cell or cell-to-matrix interactions. They act as the glue holding one cell to another cell or to the extracellular matrix. There are many CAMs that can be classified into superfamilies such as cadherins, the immunoglobulin gene superfamily (IgSF), selectins, integrins, and cell surface proteoglycans. Blood group antigens that are carried on CAMs are in Lutheran, Sc, OK, Indian, JMH, and LW systems.

The Lutheran blood groups are carried on two related red cell membrane CAMs, Lu and basal cell adhesion molecule (B-CAM). These proteins are expressed in a variety of tissues and differ only in their intracellular domains. They interact directly with spectrin, which is an integral protein in the infrastructure of the red cell membrane.

Table 14.3 Immunologically important proteins that carry blood group antigens

Red cell protein	Blood group
HLA (B7, B17, A28)	Bg^a, Bg^b, Bg^c
Complement component 4 (C4d)	Ch/Rg
Complement receptor (CR1)	Knops
Decay accelerating factor (DAF)	Cromer
Selectin	Sialyl-Le^x
Immunoglobulin superfamily (IgSF)	Lutheran, OK
Integrin (ICAM-4)	LW
CD44	Indian
Duffy antigen receptor for chemokines (DARC)	Duffy

LW (the original Rh) is an ICAM, that is, a ligand for an integrin. ICAM-4 (Inter-Cellular Adhesion Molecule), may assist in maintaining the stability of the erythroblastic islands (see below), and may be involved in removal of senescent red cells from the circulation. As part of the band 3/RhAG/Rh red cell macro-complex, ICAM-4 might also assist in facilitating transient adhesion between red cells and the vascular endothelium to maximize gas exchange. Rare individuals who lack ICAM-4 (lack LW antigens), have no apparent pathology. As its functions are critical, it is assumed that other proteins exist that compensate when ICAM-4 is missing.

Lu (BCAM, CD239) and ICAM-4, are over-expressed in red cells from patients with sickle cell disease. Lu binds to laminin (laminin is a component of the extracellular matrix abundant in basement membranes and in vascular endothelia) and ICAM-4 binds to an integrin on the endothelia of damaged blood vessels. This may contribute to blockage of vessels and painful episodes experienced by patients with sickle cell disease.

An important family of CAMs, the selectins, is responsible for the initial tethering of leukocytes to the endothelium. Adherence to the endothelium is the first step to enable leukocytes to leave the circulation and migrate into the site of tissue injury. Selectins have a long molecular structure that extends beyond the glycocalyx to capture passing leukocytes that express the appropriate receptor. Sialyl-Le^x (sLe^x) is the major ligand for selectins. Thus, sLe^x, an antigen related to the Lewis antigens, is needed for the attachment of white cells to endothelial cells. The tethering is a loose bond, because the leukocytes must be able to roll along the endothelium (like a bicycle tire on the road). ICAM-4 is involved in the integrin-mediated adherence of leukocytes to the endothelium. After this adherence, the leukocytes change shape and migrate through the endothelium. It is apparent that malignant cells move through the body (i.e. metastasize) in a similar way, and this may explain the association of sLe^x with metastases. The survival rate of sLe^x positive patients with primary liver cancer and with non-small cell lung cancer and adenocarcinoma of the colon is much lower than with sLe^x negative patients. It is conceivable that ICAM-4 is also involved in metastasis.

Yet another CAM, a cell surface proteoglycan, is CD44, which carries antigens of the Indian blood group system. This protein is present in many tissues and has a wide range of biological functions. CD44 mediates circulation of lymphocytes between blood and lymphoid organs, from which it derived its original name of "lymphocyte homing receptor". It is also involved in lymphocyte (T-cell) activation, hemopoietic development, and tumor progression and metastasis. CD44 is suppressed on red cells from individuals with the dominant type of Lutheran null phenotype. The weakened expression of the Lu glycoprotein and CD44 is caused by a nucleotide change in the *EKLF* gene, encoding a transcription factor that is necessary for efficient transcription of several genes.

Proteins involved in inflammatory response

There are associations of blood group antigens with chemokines and complement. Chemokines are members of a superfamily of chemo-attractant small proteins secreted by endothelial cells that recruit leukocytes to a site of inflammation. The chemokine receptor on red cells is the Duffy blood group glycoprotein, which is also known as the Duffy antigen receptor for chemokines (DARC). DARC is also present on endothelial cells. The function of DARC on red cells is unclear but it has been suggested that red cells act as a "sink" for clearing chemokines from the circulation. DARC is the receptor for one form of malaria merozoites.

Human Leukocyte Antigens (HLA) are sometimes found on red cells where they are considered to be remnants, left-over from their expression on immature red cells. On the red cells, HLA-B7,

HLA-B17, and HLA-A28 correspond, respectively, to Bg^a, Bg^b, and Bg^c antigens. Similarly, the weak reactions typically obtained with anti-Ch and anti-Rg are due to a breakdown product of the C4 component of complement (C4d), which is adsorbed from plasma onto circulating red cells.

Antigens of the Knops blood group system are present on the major red cell complement receptor (CR1), the receptor for complement components, C3b and C4b. CR1 is a very long protein, rather like a forsythia branch, which is freely accessible to immune complexes (soluble combinations of antigens and antibodies) that it binds and removes from the circulation.

Antigens in the Cromer blood group system are carried on decay-accelerating factor (DAF, CD55), which is an important complement regulatory protein, and a receptor for bacteria, and the picornavirus [from pico (10^{-12})—RNA—virus] (e.g. echoviruses, enteroviruses, and coxsackie viruses). DAF is present on red cells, leukocytes, platelets, and epithelial cells. The major function of DAF is to down-regulate complement activation by preventing formation of C3 and C5 convertases. DAF is anchored to the red cell membrane by a glycosylphosphaditylinositol (GPI-linked) (the protein is attached to a membrane lipid by a carbohydrate). Proteins expressing antigens in three other blood group systems (Yt, Dombrock, JMH) are also GPI-linked. This leads to another interesting association of blood groups with disease. People with a condition called Paroxysmal Nocturnal Hemoglobinuria (PNH) can have three populations of red cells with different sensitivity to complement induced lysis: PNH I red cells have normal sensitivity, PNH II red cells have a moderate sensitivity, and PNH III red cells have a marked sensitivity. PNH III red cells effectively have no GPI-linked proteins and thus lack all antigens in Yt, Dombrock, Cromer, and JMH blood group systems. If a patient with PNH has a high proportion of PNH III red cells, they will not be agglutinated by antibodies to all the antigens in these four blood group systems, so they appear like a quadruple null phenotype. While the genes for the four blood group systems are intact, the gene for attachment of GPI-linked proteins is inactive.

It seems counter intuitive for red cells to have surface adhesion molecules, because in order to perform their function, the cells need to flow freely through arteries and veins and not adhere to anything. In general, mature red cells have only a few copies of CAM molecules and young red cells express CAMs at greater density. During red cell development in the bone marrow, erythroblasts form "erythroblastic islands" around macrophages to allow the blast cell to extrude its nucleus. CAMs are needed for this adhesion. Thus, CAMs in the mature red cell membrane may be remnants from the immature red cells.

Chapter 15

The Value of Null Phenotypes

If I'd had more time, I'd have written a shorter letter.
—Mark Twain
If we'd had more time we'd have written a shorter chapter!
—Marion Reid & Ian Shine

The absence of a carbohydrate or protein carrying a blood group antigen can confer a so-called "null" (nothing) phenotype. Null phenotypes are "natural knockouts" and have revealed many secrets.

Red cell membrane

The red cell membrane is made up of three layers: an external, carbohydrate-rich layer (the glycocalyx), a lipid bilayer containing numerous transmembrane proteins, and an internal cytoplasmic network of proteins that forms the red cell membrane skeleton. Proteins carrying blood group antigens attach to the membrane in a variety of ways. Some pass through the membrane once (single pass proteins), and some pass in and out of the membrane (multipass proteins). Other proteins are attached to the outside of the cell membrane by a carbohydrate to a glycolipid (glycosylphosphaditylinositol) and these are GPI-linked proteins. (Fig. 15.1).

The mature human red cell has no nucleus and no internal organelles to repair damage, thus once released into the circulation for its three-month journey, the membrane skeleton proteins allow it to continually bend, deform, and elongate, squeezing through capillaries less than half the diameter of the red cell and then regaining its discoid shape. The unique design of the red cell and its membrane enables it to accomplish its major function of transporting respiratory gases throughout the body.

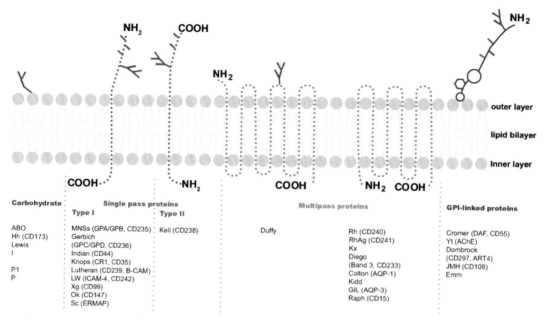

Fig. 15.1 Diagram of red cell membrane with components expressing blood group antigens

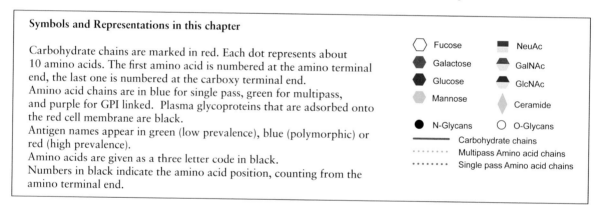

Finding null phenotypes

In general, to find people with a null phenotype by deliberate search would take an extensive effort. However, people with a null phenotype, if exposed to normal red cells through transfusion or pregnancy, will readily produce antibodies to the antigens they lack. These antibodies are easy to detect and, once identified, reveal the null phenotype. Null phenotypes have revealed insights into the role of red cell membrane proteins.

Many years of meticulous studies using agglutination assays have provided not only a vast knowledge regarding the nature of the various blood group antigens but also identified blood samples

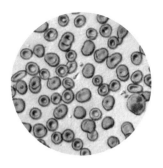

Fig. 15.2 Normocytes

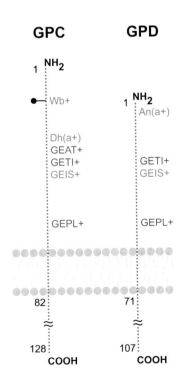

GPC   **GPD**

1 NH₂

Wb+

Dh(a+)
GEAT+
GETI+
GEIS+

1 NH₂
An(a+)

GETI+
GEIS+

GEPL+   GEPL+

82   71

128   107
COOH   **COOH**

Fig. 15.3 GPC and GPD showing the locations of some of the Gerbich antigens

with unusual characteristics for detailed genetic and molecular analysis. In turn, these genetic and molecular studies have revealed valuable information about the genes encoding the various membrane components.

The nucleotide sequence of a gene determines the amino acid sequence of the protein, from which its topology and possible function can be inferred. In general, the antigens that have significance in transfusion medicine do not alter the function of the protein. The functions predicted for carrier proteins are often based on sequence homology with proteins of known function. However, their function in the mature red cell may not be the same as in other cells. Altered forms of membrane proteins may play an important role during earlier stages of red cell development or be signals on senescent red cells.

Many red cell membrane proteins have carbohydrate structures attached to them that collectively form a negatively charged barrier, the glycocalyx, around the red cell. This barrier, which is approximately 10 to 15 nanometers deep, prevents spontaneous aggregation of red cells, and adhesion to endothelium, and may protect the red cell from invasion by microorganisms. The functions of the various red cell membrane components carrying blood group antigens can be divided into broad categories: namely, those that contribute to the integrity of the membrane structure and glycocalyx, transporters, receptors for extracellular ligands, adhesion proteins, enzymes, and complement regulatory proteins.

Null phenotype revealing a structural function

Antigens in several blood group systems are carried on proteins involved in maintaining the biconcave discoid shape of the red cell membrane (Fig. 15.2).

GERBICH BLOOD GROUPS AND ELLIPTOCYTES

The Gerbich antigens are carried on glycophorin C (GPC) and/or glycophorin D (GPD), which are glycoproteins that pass through the red cell membrane once (Fig. 15.3). The cytoplasmic domains, of GPC and GPD interact with protein 4.1R and p55 in the membrane skeleton to form a complex. The complex was shown to be important in maintaining red cell shape because individuals with Ge$_{null}$ phenotype (GPC and GPD are absent) have ellipsoid shaped red cells (Fig. 15.4).

Null Phenotypes revealing both structural and transport functions

The cell membranes are critical elements in the transport of water-soluble molecules across the hydrophobic lipid bilayer to bring in nutrients, remove waste products, and control ion gradients, thus maintaining the constancy of the internal environment.

These key functions are carried out by specialized transmembrane transport proteins that can be classified into carrier proteins that physically move a solute across the membrane, or channel proteins that form a pore in the membrane through which the specific solute or ion passes. The blood group antigen proteins for Diego, Rh, Kidd, Colton, Gill, Kx and RhAG are multipass proteins with a membrane transport function.

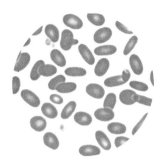

Fig. 15.4 Elliptocytes

DIEGO BLOOD GROUP SYSTEM, SPHEROCYTES, AND ANION TRANSPORT

The Diego antigens are expressed on the anion transporter (AE1, SLC4A1) also named band 3 because it is the third major band on electrophoresis. Band 3 comprises almost a third of the red cell's membrane protein; it traverses the membrane 14 times and is well anchored to the membrane skeleton through interactions with the peripheral membrane proteins, ankyrin, proteins 4.1R, and 4.2 (Fig. 15.5). In addition, band 3 plays an important role in maintaining the constancy of the internal environment; it forms

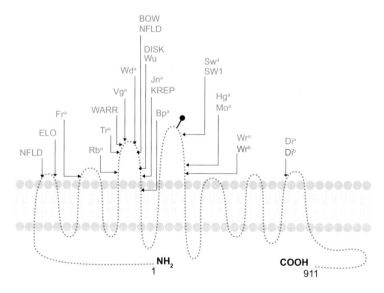

Fig. 15.5 Structure of band 3 showing the locations of the Diego antigens

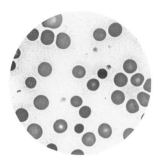

Fig. 15.6 Spherocytes

channels through the membrane that exchange bicarbonate and chloride anions, facilitating oxygen and carbon dioxide transport. The 1.2 million copies per red cell exchange approximately 20 billion bicarbonate and chloride anions per second per RBC. Band 3 also transports sulfate, phosphate, pyruvate, and superoxide, albeit at much slower rates.

In addition, the role of band 3 in maintaining red cell shape can be inferred from the effect of single amino acid substitutions in the transmembrane or the cytoplasmic domains—they are found in one fifth of patients with hereditary spherocytosis (Fig. 15.6). Other amino acid substitutions impair nephron secretion of hydrogen ions in distal renal tubular acidosis. Band 3 amino acid changes in the extracellular domain generate low prevalence blood group antigens that are not associated with pathology.

A deletion of eight amino acids of band 3 causes red cells to be elliptocytic. As this condition is found in people from Melanesia and Malasia, it is called Southeast Asian Ovalocytosis (SAO). Such red cells are unusually rigid and resist invasion by *Plasmodium falciparum* merozoites; the cells have a weakened expression of several blood group antigens, including S, s, U, En^a; D, C, e; Kp^b; Jk^a, Jk^b; Di^b, Wr^b; Xg^a; Sc1; IF and IT. No homozygote has been found, suggesting it is lethal. Only one person has been described with the Diego$_{null}$ phenotype. To survive his hemolytic anemia, he required life-long transfusions.

In addition to these functions, band 3 also may be involved in removal of damaged or senescent red cells from the circulation. As the red cell ages, events trigger band 3 to cluster, thereby generating a signal that is recognized by IgG antibodies in the plasma. The bound antibody then acts as a signal for phagocytes to remove aged or defective red cells from the circulation.

RH BLOOD GROUP SYSTEM, STOMATOCYTES, AND GAS TRANSPORT

Antigens in the Rh blood group system are expressed by two homologous proteins: RhD, and RhCE. Rh antigen expression at the red cell surface requires the presence of a related protein, the Rh-associated glycoprotein (RhAG). RhD, RhCE and RhAG, (Fig. 15.7), together with LW glycoprotein, integrin-associated protein (IAP, CD47), glycophorin B and possibly Duffy protein, form a core complex in the red cell membrane. This core complex transports NH_4^+/NH_3 and CO_2/O_2 or cation across the membrane.

The importance of the Rh complex in regulating red cell membrane structure was revealed by the rare Rh$_{null}$ phenotype, because the red cells are stomatocytes (*stoma* Greek for mouth, *kytos* Greek for vessel) (Fig. 15.8). Rh$_{null}$ red cells have a shortened survival, leading to a compensated hemolytic anemia.

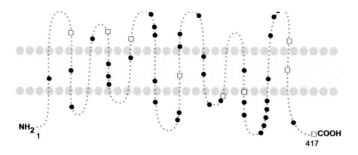
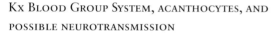

Fig. 15.7 RhD, RhCE and RhAG are predicted to pass through the red cell membrane 12 times. The rectangles mark the junctions of amino acids encoded by the 10 exons. The ● (black circles) indicate the amino acids that differ between RhD and RhCE

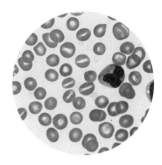

Fig. 15.8 Stomatocytes

KX BLOOD GROUP SYSTEM, ACANTHOCYTES, AND POSSIBLE NEUROTRANSMISSION

A gene on the short arm of the X chromosome encodes the Kx antigen that is expressed on the XK protein (Fig. 15.9). The structural similarity with transporters of neurotransmitters across neuron membranes suggests XK is a membrane transport protein.

The high prevalence antigen Kx is inherited as an X linked recessive. The absence of the antigen is associated with an interesting phenotype named after Hugh McLeod, a Harvard dental student who donated blood in 1961. Before the unit was used it was found to be hemolysing, it contained many acanthocytes and reacted weakly with Kell antibodies (see p. 76).

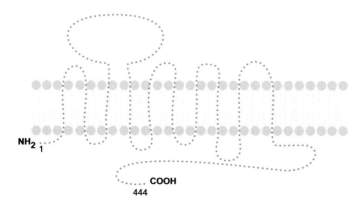

Fig. 15.9 XK protein

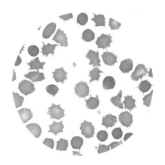

Fig. 15.10 Acanthocytes

People with this rare syndrome (all males) have 8% to 85% acanthocytes (Fig. 15.10), a mild, compensated hemolytic anemia, elevated levels of serum creatine phosphokinase and carbonic anhydrase, late (after 40) onset muscular dystrophy, cardiomyopathy, and peripheral neuropathy. Red cell survival is reduced. Clinically there may be progressive choreiform movements and dystonia and areflexia. The acanthocytosis can be corrected with chlorpromazine, which expands the cytoplasmic leaflet of the red cell bilayer, thus promoting inward curvature. Female heterozygotes do not have muscle or neurological diseases but they have occasional acanthocytes, as expected with X-chromosome inactivation.

Null phenotypes revealing transport functions

Other proteins carrying blood group antigens (Kidd, Colton, and Gill) also pass through the lipid bilayer many times and function as transporters but do not appear to be involved in membrane structure or red cell shape (Table 15.1).

KIDD BLOOD GROUP SYSTEM AND TRANSPORT OF UREA

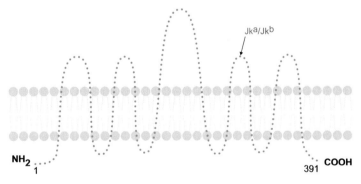

Fig. 15.11 Structure of Kidd glycoprotein

Antigens of the Kidd blood group system are expressed on the Kidd glycoprotein, also known as the urea transporter (Fig. 15.11). The rare Jk_{null} phenotype is found more frequently in Polynesians and Finns than in other populations. The observation that Jk_{null} cells were relatively resistant to lysis by 2M urea provided the clue that the Kidd glycoprotein transports urea. Red cells rapidly transport urea across their membrane as they pass through the high urea concentration in the renal medulla, and thereby prevent red cell dehydration. Urea transport across Jk_{null} red cell membranes is approximately a

Table 15.1 The function and tissue distribution of blood group systems and the disease associations with null phenotypes

Function	System name	Present in other tissue	Null Phenotype	Disease association
Structure and function				
Membrane attachment; interacts with protein 4.1R and p55	GE	Fetal liver, renal endothelium, brain, cerebellum, ilium	Leach	Hereditary Elliptocytosis, hemolytic anemia.
Anion exchanger	DI	Granulocytes, kidney: intercalated cells of distal and collecting tubules, testes	1 case –transfusion dependent	Southeast Asian Ovalocytosis, Hereditary Spherocytosis, Renal tubular acidosis
NH_4+/ NH_3 and CO_2/ O_2 or cation	RHAG	Kidney, central nervous system	Rh_{null}	Hemolytic anemia, hereditary stomatocytosis, hematological malignancies
Possible neurotransmitter	KX	Fetal liver, adult skeletal muscle, brain, pancreas, heart	McLeod	Acanthocytosis, muscular dystrophy, hemolytic anemia, (McLeod syndrome)
Transport				
Urea transporter	JK	Vasa recta endothelium Renal medulla vascular supply	Jk(a–b–)	Impaired urea transport, urine concentrating defect
Water channel	CO	Kidney, liver, lung, gall bladder, eye, capillary endothelium	Co(a–b–)	Monosomy 7, congenital dyserythropoietic anemia Anoxia and angiogenesis
Glycerol/ water/urea transport	GIL	Kidney, liver, pancreas, lung, spleen, prostate	GIL-negative	

thousand times slower than across normal red cell membranes. No changes in either red cell shape or life-span have been noted in association with absence of Kidd glycoprotein. Patients with Jk_{null} red cells have an impaired ability to maximally concentrate urine.

Colton blood group system and transport of water

Antigens in the Colton blood group system are carried on the Colton glycoprotein, which was discovered and named aquaporin-1 (AQP-1) (Fig. 15.12) by Peter Agre[1] in 1992.

AQP-1 is a tetramer, forming an hour glass structure 2.75 Angstroms wide, so finely adjusted that water molecules, also 2.75 Angstroms wide, pass through it in single file. Amazing! It is the water channel in many tissues of many animals and many plants.

The body makes 2.4 million red cells every second; each red cell membrane contains 200,000 AQP-1 water channels. The AQP-1 unit permeability was $\sim 3 \times 10^9$ water molecules per subunit per second.

1. Despite having an idyllic childhood and a father who was a PhD chemist and whose family friends included Linus Pauling, Peter Agre was not a perfect student. When he obtained a D grade in chemistry he withdrew from high school. But he went on to medical school at Johns Hopkins, and clinical studies at Case Western University Hospital in Cleveland.

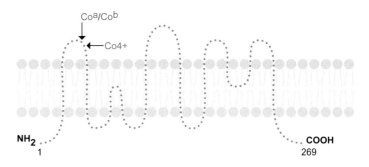

Fig. 15.12 Structure of Colton glycoprotein

Using membrane analytical techniques learned at University of North Carolina, Agre discovered severe spectrin deficiency in two children with severe spherocytosis. Victor McKusick helped him return to Hopkins where he set up a laboratory where he began to determine the structure of the Rh polypeptide. He found a persistent, novel 28 kDa protein that he thought might be part of the Rh molecule, or a contaminant. A similar protein was known in many species and in many diverse tissues, being especially abundant in the descending loop of Henle and the proximal renal tubules. John Parker at Chapel Hill suggested that it might be the elusive water channel that had been long predicted. Agre demonstrated that cells containing this protein swelled by osmosis, those lacking the protein did not. He then inserted the protein into artificial cells making them permeable. He determined its structure and identified the structural gene for aquaporin-1 (AQP-1 was as part of the Colton blood group on chromosome 7. This discovery led to Peter Agre winning a Nobel Prize in Chemistry in 2003, that he attributed to serendipity, fine collaborators and valuable advice that he generously acknowledged.

Equilibrium is achieved in 30 ms and the driving force is simply osmosis.

Under normal physiological conditions, the high membrane permeability of red cells facilitates the rapid rehydration of red cells after their shrinkage in the hypertonic environment of the renal medulla. Quite reasonably, it was thought that an absence of AQP-1 would be incompatible with life. However, the identification of an antibody to a high prevalence antigen by serologists revealed extremely rare Co_{null} individuals whose red cells lack AQP-1. They exhibit markedly reduced osmotic permeability, defective urinary concentrating ability as well as decreased pulmonary vascular permeability but they are apparently healthy.

Knock out mice have demonstrated aquaporin control of water movement into and out of the brain, and also an influence on cell migration, angiogenesis, tumor metastasis, wound healing, sensory signaling and seizures.

GIL BLOOD GROUP SYSTEM AND TRANSPORT OF GLYCEROL, WATER AND UREA

The blood group antigen, GIL, was shown to be expressed on aquaporin-3 (AQP-3) by studying two individuals whose plasma contained antibodies to this high prevalence antigen (Fig. 15.13).

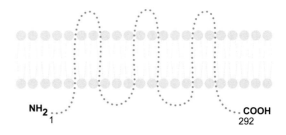

Fig. 15.13 Structure of GIL glycoprotein

Like AQP-1, AQP-3 is also a MIP channel-forming molecule, but differs from AQP-1 in that, in addition to water, it also transports other small non-ionic molecules such as glycerol and urea. Studies on glycerol permeability in AQP-3 deficient red cells (GIL_{null}) led to the proposal that another protein is also involved in the transport of glycerol. The observations are consistent with the fact that GIL_{null} red cells are not associated with any overt functional defect. AQP-3 traverses the red cell membrane six times. APQ-3 is expressed in other tissues including, kidney, liver, pancreas, lung, spleen, and prostate. AQP-3 is important in regulating epidermal structure and function.

Null phenotypes revealing membrane proteins that act as receptors for parasites, bacteria, and viruses

Based on their structure or function in other cells, some proteins in the red cell membrane that carry blood group antigens appear to be receptors for specific ligands or microorganisms, suggesting the components may play a direct role in the pathogenesis of infectious diseases (Table 15.2).

DUFFY BLOOD GROUP SYSTEM AND MALARIA

As summarized in Chapter 14, antigens of the Duffy blood group system are, logically enough, carried on the Duffy glycoprotein. Although the Duffy glycoprotein is predicted to have seven membrane-spanning domains (Fig. 15.14), it has not been shown to transport molecules across the membrane.

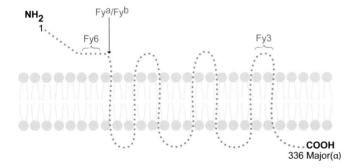

Fig. 15.14 Structure of Duffy glycoprotein

The Duffy glycoprotein is a promiscuous chemokine receptor in red cells that binds pro-inflammatory cytokines of both the C-X-C

Table 15.2 Tissue distribution and disease association for some proteins carrying blood group systems with receptor or adhesion function

Function	System name	Present in other tissue	Null Phenotype	Disease association
Chemokine/ *Plasmodium vivax* receptor	FY	Endothelial, and epithelial cells, Purkinje cells of cerebellum, colon, lung, spleen, thyroid, thymus, collecting ducts of kidney	Fy(a–b–)	The null are resistance to *P vivax* invasion
Binds hyaluronic acid, mediates adhesion of leukocytes	IN	Wide tissue distribution	1 case of Congenital Dyserythropoietic anemia	Depressed in pregnancy
Binds integrins to laminin and collagen	RAPH	Fibroblasts, kidney, skin, inner ear	MER2–	Hereditary nephritis, epidermolysis bullosa, neurosensory deafness.
Binds laminin	LU	Fetal liver, placenta, arterial walls, bone marrow, epithelium	Lu(a–b–) recessive type	Increased expression possibly involved in vaso-occlusion in sickle cell disease
Binds CD11/CD18. Ligand for integrins	LW	Blood cells, epidermis, the blood/brain barrier	LW_{null} also Rh_{null}	Depressed in pregnancy and in some malignant diseases. More strongly expressed on neonatal RBCs
Possible adhesion signal transduction	OK	All cells tested	Not described	Tumor growth factor Tumor genesis
Adhesion molecule	XG	Fibroblasts, fetal liver, spleen, thymus, adrenal, adult bone marrow	Not described	
Adhesion molecule. Function in RBCs not known	JMH	Activated lymphocytes, neurons, epithelia and testes	Not described	Absent from PNH III RBCs
Possible adhesion	SC	Erythroid specific	Sc:–1,–2,–3	
Binds microbes; contributes to the glycocalyx; complement regulation; chaperone for band 3	MNS	Renal endothelium and epithelium	M^kM^k (lack GPA & GPB) En(a–) (lack GPA) S–s– (lack GPB)	Decreased *P. falciparum* invasion. May be receptor for some strains of *E. coli* and for influenza virus

133

class (acute inflammation) and the C-C class (chronic inflammation), including IL-8, MGSA (melanoma growth stimulatory activity), MCP-1 (monocyte chemotactic protein 1) and RANTES (regulated on activation, normal T-expressed and secreted). This chemokine receptor role was revealed by testing red cells with the Fy_{null} [Fy(a–b–)] phenotype, which also revealed that the Duffy glycoprotein is the receptor for the malarial parasite, *Plasmodium vivax* (Fig. 15.15).

In 1955, Race and Sanger were surprised to observe that the Fy_{null} phenotype, which is rare in most populations, is the predominant phenotype among African populations, particularly those originating in West Africa, where the incidence of Fy_{null} may reach 100%. During the same year, it was reported that a majority of Africans were resistant to *Plasmodium vivax*. Malaria was originally thought to be caused by the poisonous emanations (miasma) of the bad air (malària) near swamps until, in 1897, Ross recognized that it was caused by a parasite transmitted by female anopheles mosquitoes that lay their eggs in stagnant water. In 1977, Louis Miller and others showed that of 17 volunteers who were exposed to *P. vivax* infected mosquitoes, the 5 Fy_{null} subjects were the only ones who did not develop malaria. Although *P. vivax* has a lower mortality than *P. falciparum*, it is a large burden, with over 80 million cases a year out of about 300 million cases of all types of malaria (Fig. 15.16).

Because Fy_{null} red cells are refractory to invasion by *P. vivax* merozoites, it is likely that this phenotype, at least in Africa, is at a selective advantage. However, a small number of people with the Fy_{null} phenotype have recently contracted *P. vivax* malaria. Thus, it appears that the parasite has mutated, which is disturbing.

The lack of Duffy glycoprotein in red cells from Africans is the result of a nucleotide change in the promoter region of the gene encoding the Duffy glycoprotein. This disrupts a binding site for the erythroid transcription factor GATA-1 and prevents expression of the Duffy gene in erythroid cells, but not on non-erythroid tissues.

Rare individuals with the "true" Fy_{null} phenotype, that is, they lack the Duffy glycoprotein not only from red cells but from all tissues, have no obvious hematological or immunological abnormalities.

MNS BLOOD GROUP SYSTEM AND GLYCOPHORIN A (GPA) AND GLYCOPHORIN B (GPB) AND MALARIA

GPA and GPB (Fig. 15.17), which express antigens in the MNS blood group system, are single pass membrane glycoproteins that account for the majority of the surface charge of the red cell.

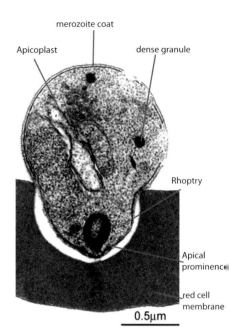

Fig. 15.15 A merozoite in the process of invading an RBC

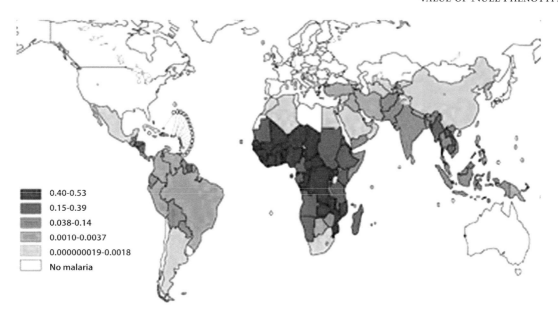

Fig. 15.16 The World Distribution of all types of malaria showing prevalence measured as suspected number of cases by total population per year. For example, in 2009 there were 2.6 million suspected cases in Brazil with a population of 193 million (1.3 per cent), and 3 million out of 13 million in Zambia (23 per cent). Worldwide there are about one million deaths per annum.

2. The discovery of the molecular basis of MN antigens

In the late 1960s, little was known about the structure of the red cell membrane. The thinking was that the membrane consists of a single protein, like collagen. Dr Vincent Marchesi and his team at Yale University, and Dr Olga Blumenfeld with one technologist at the Albert Einstein Medical School in New York, independently determined the amino acid sequence of the glycophorin. An important aspect of the purification procedure was that it had become possible to isolate a sufficient quantity of pure protein (20 mg) for chemical analysis from one unit of blood (450 mL). By 1978, Marchesi had obtained the full amino acid sequence, determined the carbohydrate attachment sites, and the disposition within the membrane of a glycoprotein

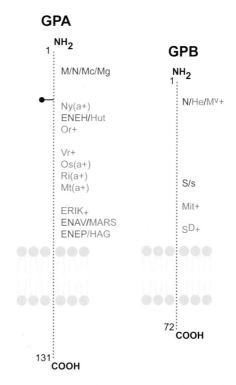

Fig. 15.17 Structure of GPA and GPB showing location of antigens due to simple amino acid changes. The gene encoding GPB (*GYPB*) arose from *GYPA* by gene duplication.

Their extracellular domains contain an abundance of sialic acid, which contributes to the layer of negative charge at the cell surface, preventing adherence of red cells to each other and to the vessel walls. The carbohydrate component of GPA accounts for two thirds of its molecular mass. GPA was the first membrane protein to have its complete amino acid sequence determined.[2] GPA also serves as a receptor for certain microorganisms, such as *E. coli*, influenza virus and *P. falciparum*, and may function as a chaperone, facilitating the targeting of specific proteins, such as band 3, to the membrane.

Band 3 & glycophorin A are functionally associated

GPA and band 3 have a physiologically relevant association. The expression of the Wr[b] blood group antigen requires the interaction between amino acids 59–72 on GPA and Glu658 on band 3. Indeed, the GPA Ala65 to Pro variant (HAG antigen) and the Glu63 to Lys variant (MARS antigen) cause weakened Wr[b] antigen expression. The sugars on GPA are an attachment site for *P. falciparum*. There are alternative pathways for malarial invasion of red cells that depend on the strain of *P. falciparum* and the ability of the parasite to switch its invasion requirements. For example, sialic acid-dependent invasion results from binding of merozoite protein EBA-175 to the sialic acid-galactose disaccharide on the O-linked tetrasaccharides of GPA. Another sialic acid-dependent but EBA-175 independent pathway is believed to involve merozoite binding to GPB.

Rare humans have a deletion of gene(s) that causes a complete loss of GPA, or GPB, or both, which gives rise, respectively, to En(a–), S–s–, and M[k]M[k] red cells. En(a–) red cells, for example, are completely deficient in GPA. The affected red cells compensate for a loss of surface charge by increasing the glycosylation of band 3, such that the overall surface charge is only reduced by 20%. None of the GPA and GPB variants produce detectable changes in the shape, function, or life-span of the affected red cells. GPA binds the C4 component of complement and may provide limited protection to red cells from complement-induced lysis by inhibiting the formation or binding of the C5b-C7 complex.

they named "glycophorin" (GPA). The pure glycoprotein isolated by Blumenfeld was also glycophorin A, which in 1971 Dr C. Howe at Columbia University demonstrated had M and N activity.

Together with Philip Levine, Dr Blumenfeld recognized that the amino terminal peptide of her extract contained equimolar amounts: one sequence corresponded to M and the other to N; the donor was M+N+. Blumenfeld then found a threonine to asparagine substitution in the amino terminal domain of GPA associated with the Mg antigen that Dr M.N. Metaxas had provided. Simultaneously, Marchesi and H. Furthmayr sequenced two variants: Mg and Mc. Using a clone generously provided by Minoru Fukuda in La Jolla, California, Blumenfeld analyzed the gene encoding GPA. She assigned Dr Cheng-Han Huang to study glycophorin variants. They identified a deletion of the glycophorin B gene (the S–s–U– phenotype), one of the first for which the molecular basis became known. Thereafter, many other investigators determined the molecular basis of numerous blood group antigens. Following this success, in 1998 Blumenfeld started, and has since maintained, a database (dbRBC) for variant blood group alleles. This database is now curated by NCBI.

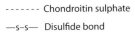
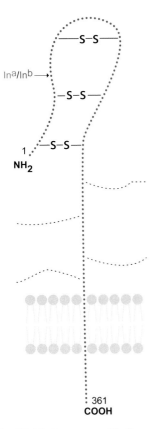

NH$_2$
1

361
COOH

Fig. 15.18 Structure of Indian glycoprotein (CD44)

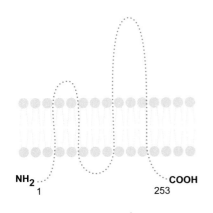

NH$_2$
1

COOH
253

Fig. 15.19 Structure of CD151

Null phenotypes revealing membrane proteins that act as adhesion proteins

Cell adhesion molecules are crucial for many normal physiological processes in embryogenesis, as well as in processes such as inflammation, wound healing, and cancer. Although adhesion molecules have no obvious function on mature red cells, they are likely to play a key role in cell-to-cell or cell-matrix interaction during erythropoiesis.

Indian blood group system

Antigens of the Indian system are carried on CD44, a single pass membrane protein (Fig. 15.18). CD44 may be the major receptor for hyaluronic acid, a large molecule that is widespread in the body. It may also bind fibrinogen, laminin, some forms of collagen, and osteopontin. CD44-hyaluronan interaction may be required for adhesion of lymphoid cells and erythrocyte burst-forming units to bone marrow stroma in lymphopoiesis and erythropoiesis.

Isoforms of CD44, as a consequence of alternative splicing, are associated with the ability of cancer cells to metastasize. Soluble forms of CD44 have been found in plasma of cancer patients and in non-Hodgkin's lymphoma; a correlation between clinical severity and CD44 levels was observed. The In(a–b–) phenotype was described in a patient with a novel form of congenital dyserythropoietic anemia (CDA) and CD44 deficiency but it was not possible to determine if the phenotype was genetic or related to the patient's hematological disorder. The red cells of the patient also typed AnWj–, and Co(a–b–). The anemia is now known to be due to a mutation in the X-linked GATA-1 gene, which encodes a transcription factor.

RAPH blood group system

MER2 is the only antigen of the RAPH blood group system (named after Raphael, the first name of the first patient whose plasma contained anti-MER2). It is of no clinical significance in transfusion medicine, yet its study has shed light on the importance of a protein, CD151 (Fig. 15.19), in the maintenance of stability of basement membranes. One healthy Turkish blood donor and three sick Israelis of Indian-Jewish ancestry were described with the RAPH$_{null}$ phenotype. The three have hereditary nephritis leading to end-stage renal failure, neurosensory deafness and pretibial epidermolysis bullosa. CD151 is a member of the tetraspanin superfamily (so named because it spans the membrane four times).

Tetraspanins in the cell membrane aggregate with each other and with a variety of other transmembrane proteins, in particular integrins, and transmembrane receptors involved in adhesion and cell-signaling. CD151 appears to function as a link between integrins and the extracellular matrix glycoproteins laminin and collagen in kidney and skin. The RAPH$_{null}$ patients have abnormal basement membranes in the kidney, which gives rise to their hereditary nephritis, and in the skin, which is responsible for their epidermolysis bullosa, and, possibly, in the inner ear, hence their neurosensory deafness.

Immunoglobulin-superfamily of glycoproteins

At least six proteins in the red cell membrane belong to the immunoglobulin superfamily (IgSF) of glycoproteins. Four carry blood group antigens in Lutheran, LW, Scianna or Ok systems, and two, CD47 and CD58, do not express blood group antigens. The IgSF glycoproteins primarily function as receptors and adhesion molecules.

Lutheran Blood Group System

The Lutheran blood group glycoprotein (Fig. 15.20) is the receptor on erythroid cells for the extracellular matrix protein, laminin. The glycoprotein consists of five disulfide-bonded extracellular, IgSF domains, a single hydrophobic transmembrane domain and a cytoplasmic tail. Two isoforms of this single pass membrane protein [85 kilodaltons (Lu) and 78 kilodaltons (B-CAM)] are expressed by alternative splicing of a single gene. Both isoforms bind laminin. The two isoforms are distinguished by differences in their cytoplasmic domains—the 78 kilodalton isoform has a truncated cytoplasmic tail (B-CAM). While the function of the Lutheran glycoprotein in normal red cells remains to be defined, it mediates adhesion of red cells with sickle hemoglobin (HbSS) to laminin. Red cells from patients with sickle cell disease express approximately one and a half times more Lutheran glycoprotein than normal red cells and the level of laminin binding to red cells correlates with the level of Lutheran expression.

As Lutheran glycoprotein is expressed late during erythroid differentiation, it has been suggested that it may play a role in mediating erythroblast-extracellular matrix interactions in the bone marrow that regulate egress of reticulocytes from the bone

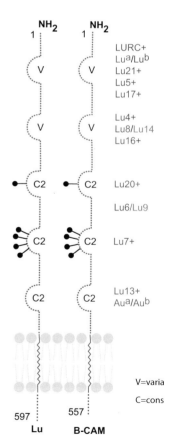

Fig. 15.20 Structure of Lutheran and B-CAM glycoprotein

3. Mary (Polly) Crawford was trained as a pediatrician but found her deafness too big a hurdle to use the stethoscope effectively. She turned her talented hands and mind to transfusion medicine. After her husband died, she established the Pearson C. Cummin Memorial Laboratory in the basement of her home. Polly was a skilled bird-watcher and popular among colleagues because she had a rare blood type. She phenotyped her own red cells and was surprised when they were not agglutinated by the only example of anti-Lu[b] that she had in her inventory. When she visited Tibi Greenwalt at the Milwaukee Blood Center, who had found the second example of anti-Lu[b], presuming her red cells were the rare Lu(a+b–) type, she offered to give him a blood sample. Surprisingly, Polly's red cells typed Lu(a–)! Race and Sanger confirmed the typing. Polly was the first example of the rare Lu(a–b–) phenotype.

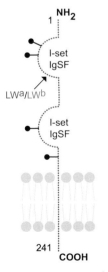

Fig. 15.21 Structure of LW glycoprotein (ICAM-4)

marrow into the circulation.

The cytoplasmic region of Lutheran glycoprotein interacts with the membrane skeleton. Three genetic backgrounds generate the Lu(a–b–) phenotype: (i) homozygosity for a recessive autosomal gene *LU*, (ii) a dominant suppressor gene *InLu* (*ELFK*), and (iii) an X-linked recessive gene (*GATA-1*). Only the autosomal recessive type of Lu(a–b–) can be considered a true null phenotype because weak expression of Lutheran antigens can be demonstrated for the two other types. There is no obvious disease implication associated with a lack of the Lu glycoproteins. It is of interest for three reasons. The *InLu* gene (*EKLF*) product has broad regulatory powers. It inhibits expression of CD44 (an adhesive protein carrying the Indian blood group), CD151 (a protein carrying the MER2 antigen), CR1 (the C3b/C4b complement receptor carrying the Knops blood group), AnWj (the erythroid *Haemophilus influenzae* receptor), and the glycolipid antigens P1 and i, as well as the Lutheran antigens. Second, although some of these proteins (e.g., CD44) are widely expressed, the action of *In(Lu)* is limited to erythroid cells. Third, some patients with the InLu Lu(a–b–) phenotype have red cells that vary from normocytes to acanthocytes. No hemolysis or anemia is evident in these people. Osmotic fragility of fresh dominant Lu(a–b–) red cells is normal but, during incubation, the red cells lose potassium ions and lyse more readily than normal red cells. This phenomenon was noted by Polly Crawford[3], whose own red cells were of the dominant Lu(a–b–) phenotype.

LW BLOOD GROUP SYSTEM

The LW glycoprotein [intracellular adhesion molecule-4 (ICAM-4)] (Fig. 15.21) consists of two extracellular IgSF domains, which show strong sequence homology with the protein superfamily of intracellular adhesion molecules (ICAMs). Extracellular domains of LW glycoprotein interact with certain integrins. In contrast to Lutheran glycoprotein, which is expressed late during erythroid development, LW glycoprotein is expressed early during erythropoiesis before GPA and about the same time as RhAG. It has been suggested that LW glycoprotein may play a role in erythroblast-macrophage interactions in erythroblastic islands, which are critical for erythropoiesis.

The proband (Mrs Big) and her brother who have the rare inherited LW$_{null}$ phenotype, are apparently normal. Transient loss of LW antigen from the red cells has been reported in pregnancy and with lymphoma, leukemia, sarcoma, and other forms of malignancy, and could represent some underlying immunological disorder.

The LW protein is part of the Rh complex and is expressed on D-negative red cells at about half the number as is present in D-positive red cells. In cord blood samples the number of copies of LW glycoprotein per red cell is equal in D-positive and D-negative red cells and is higher than in D-positive adults. The reason for this is unknown.

Ok Blood Group System

The red cell antigen, Ok^a, is located on the Ok glycoprotein, a leukocyte activation antigen with two IgSF domains. The function of the Ok glycoprotein (synonym CD147, neurothelin, basigin) (Fig.15.22) in red cells is unknown although sequence homologies within the cytoplasmic and transmembrane domains suggest that it could be a component of a signal transduction complex.

The Ok^a antigen occurs with a high prevalence and the few Ok(a–) probands have been Japanese.

Scianna Blood Group System

Human erythrocyte membrane associated protein (ERMAP, Fig. 15.23) is expressed exclusively on erythroid cells and carries Scianna antigens. ERMAP is predicted to have one extracellular transmembrane Ig-like domain. The intracellular region has a conserved B30.2 domain and multiple kinase-dependent phosphorylation consensus motifs. ERMAP is likely to be a signal transduction molecule specific for red cells. People with the null phenotype are apparently normal. Several such people are Marshall islanders.

Xg Blood Group System

The Xg glycoprotein (Fig. 15.24) is homologous with CD99, which has adhesion properties. It can mediate apoptosis and is thought to be important in hemopoietic cell differentiation. The function of Xg glycoprotein in red cells is not known.

The difference between the Xg(a+) and Xg(a–) phenotype is associated with the expression level of the Xg^a antigen and, presumably, Xg glycoprotein on the red cell surface rather than a variant gene product. Xg^a antigen escapes X-chromosome inactivation due to its localization partially within the pseudoautosomal region of the X chromosome (Fig. 15.25).

CD99 (MIC2) is expressed ubiquitously and is an adhesion molecule on T cells. A portion of CD99 activates a caspase independent apoptosis pathway in T-cells.

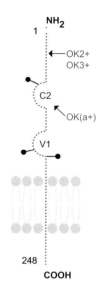

Fig. 15.22 Structure of Ok glycoprotein (CD147)

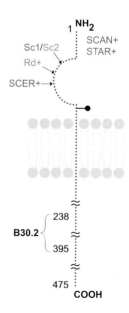

Fig. 15.23 Structure of ERMAP showing location of Scianna antigens

Fig. 15.24 Xg glycoprotein

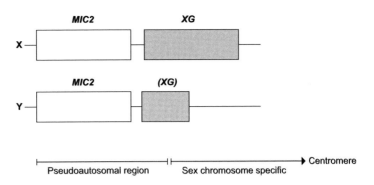

Fig. 15.25 Pseudo-autosomal region of X and Y chromosome

JMH BLOOD GROUP SYSTEM

The JMH antigen is carried on the GPI-linked protein CD108 (Fig. 15.26) expressed on red cells, some activated lymphocytes, neurons, epithelia and testes. CD108 molecules are part of plasma membrane complexes that are associated with intracellular protein kinases. Like other GPI-linked molecules, CD108 on red cells and other cells may be a receptor that plays a role in signal transduction.

Null phenotypes revealing membrane proteins that function as enzymes

KELL BLOOD GROUP SYSTEM

The Kell glycoprotein (Fig. 15.27) is a single pass membrane protein that is firmly attached by a covalent bond to the multipass protein, Xk (Fig.15.9). Kell glycoprotein has sequence homology with a family of neutral endopeptidases and is an endothelin-3 converting enzyme. Endothelins are potent vasoactive peptides involved both in the regulation of vascular tone and in developmental processes by affecting differentiation of neural-crest-derived cells. The Kell glycoprotein may participate in the early stages of hemopoiesis or cell lineage determination. Kell deficient red cells are normal.

The antigens in the Kell blood group system are each associated with a single amino acid substitution of the Kell glycoprotein. The k to K substitution of threonine to methionine disrupts the motif (Asn-X-Thr [where X represents any amino acid other than proline]) for N-glycosylation. The absence of the sugar may expose the K antigen and explain the immunogenicity of this antigen.

Like anti-D, anti-K causes HDN. In addition to triggering anemia by the premature removal of antibody-coated fetal red

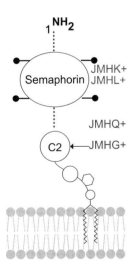

Fig. 15.26 Structure of JMH glycoprotein (CD108)

cells, anti-K also suppresses erythropoiesis. This produces an even more profound anemia than caused by anti-D. Because of the suppression of erythropoieses, the strength of anti-K in maternal plasma cannot be used as an indicator of how severely a fetus is affected by HDN.

YT BLOOD GROUP SYSTEM

Yt antigens reside on acetylcholinesterase (AChE). In red cells, AChE (Fig. 15.28) is GPI-linked and it resides in the membrane as a dimer. Its function in red cells is not known but the molecule is enzymatically active and the Yt^a/Yt^b polymorphism (which results from a single amino acid substitution) does not affect the enzymatic activity of AChE.

On nerve cells, AChE is a conventional single pass transmembrane protein, likely arising from alternative splicing of the mRNA.

DOMBROCK BLOOD GROUP SYSTEM

The Dombrock antigens reside on ADP-ribosyltransferase, another GPI-linked glycoprotein (Fig. 15.29). This enzyme (ART4) acts as a regulator of protein function through post-translational modification of the addition of ADP-ribose to a target molecule. Despite extensive investigation, the red cell Dombrock glycoprotein has not yet been shown to have enzymatic activity. Red cells with the Do_{null} phenotype have normal structure and function.

Null phenotypes revealing membrane proteins with functions of complement elements and regulation

CROMER BLOOD GROUP SYSTEM

Antigens in the Cromer blood group system are located on decay accelerating factor (DAF, CD55, Fig. 15.30), which is attached to the red cell membrane through a GPI-anchor. The DAF glycoprotein is arranged into four extracellular complement control protein (CCP) domains, each with about 60 amino acid residues.

DAF is present on all cells that are in contact with plasma (including blood cells and vascular endothelium), on epithelia of the gastrointestinal and urinary tracts, and in the nervous system. DAF is strongly expressed on the apical surface of trophoblasts.

It will absorb antibodies to antigens in the Cromer system, from maternal plasma, thereby explaining why Cromer incompatibility

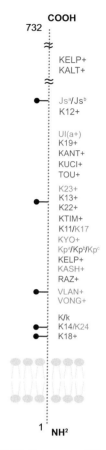

Fig. 15.27 Structure of Kell glycoprotein (CD238) showing location of Kell antigens

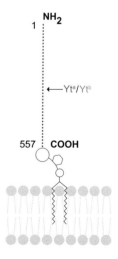

Fig. 15.28 Structure of AChE showing location of Yt^a/Yt^b antigens

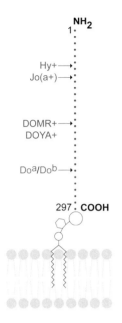

Fig. 15.29 Structure of Dombrock glycoprotein (CD297) showing location of antigens

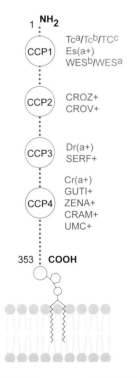

Fig. 15.30 Structure of DAF (CD55) showing location of Cromer antigens

does not cause HDN. It was thought that DAF was the cause of susceptibility of PNH III red cells to lysis; however, the finding of the Cromer$_{null}$ phenotype (also called the Inab phenotype after the first proband, Inaba, who was Japanese) revealed that DAF is not the primary cause. Other membrane proteins are also involved in this susceptibility to lysis.

DAF accelerates the decay of both C3 and C5 convertases, regardless of whether they are the products of the classical or alternative pathways of complement activation. Thus, DAF inhibits the amplification of complement and protects cells from lysis. DAF is a receptor for *E. coli* and for enterovirus.

Red cells from individuals with the Cromer$_{null}$ phenotype do not have significant complement-induced lysis in vivo. However, protein-loosing enteropathy and other gut abnormalities have been reported for several people with this Inab phenotype.

KNOPS BLOOD GROUP SYSTEM

Like the gene encoding DAF, the CR1 gene is located within the regulation of complement activation cluster on chromosome 1q32. Antigens of the Knops system are carried on complement receptor 1 (CR1; CD35). CR1 is a single pass membrane glycoprotein (Fig. 15.31) and a member of the CCP family. The CR1 glycoprotein consists of up to 30 repeated, and disulfide-bonded, CCP domains. These repeat domains are organized into four regions called long homologous repeats (LHRs), each region consisting of seven CCPs. Knops antigen expression is variable among different individuals, as is the number of CR1 molecules per red cell. CR1 protects red cells from autohemolysis by inhibiting the classical and alternative complement pathways through cleavage of C4b and C3b.

Acquired deficiencies of CR1 have been described in patients with systemic lupus erythematosus, rheumatic diseases, malignancies, and inflammatory disorders. Low levels of CR1 on red cells may cause deposition of immune complexes on blood vessel walls with subsequent damage to the vessels.

In laboratory tests, the ability of *P. falciparum* to attach to uninfected red cells (rosetting) is reduced in those with a Knops variant [Sl(a−)] or that have a low CR1 level. This suggests that the Sl(a−) phenotype confers resistance to malaria caused by *P. falciparum*. The Sl(a−) phenotype is more common in Africans and may have developed as a protective mechanism. The antigens to the Knops blood group system are carried on CCPs 22, 24 and 25.

Other null phenotypes

Most of the remaining components expressing blood group antigens are carbohydrates and are involved in forming the glycocalyx and/or are adsorbed from the plasma (Table 15.3).

CHIDO/RODGERS BLOOD GROUP SYSTEM

The complement elements C4A and C4B carry, respectively, the Rodgers and Chido antigens and are adsorbed by red cells from the plasma. C4 (Fig. 15.32) is involved in complement activation by the classical pathway. Functionally, C4A is more effective than C4B in breaking down immune complexes and inhibiting immune precipitation. C4B binds more efficiently to the red cells, thus causing lysis.

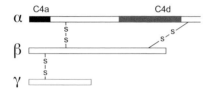

Fig. 15.32 Structure of C4

Of eighteen cases with total C4 deficiency (Ch/Rg$_{null}$), 14 had systemic lupus erythematosus. C4A$_{null}$ has been associated with numerous other autoimmune diseases, for example Graves' disease, rheumatoid arthritis, and Sjörgen syndrome. C4B$_{null}$ has been associated with IgA nephropathy, rheumatoid arthritis, and increased susceptibility to bacterial meningitis in children.

A, B, H AND LEWIS BLOOD GROUP SYSTEM

The ABO antigens (Fig. 15.33) require the sequential action of glycosyltransferases for expression. Lack of A, B and H antigens on red cells, as in individuals with the Bombay (O$_h$) phenotype, does not affect red cell function, integrity or survival and there are no reports of increased propensity to infection or disease in these individuals.

The carbohydrate antigens A, B, H, Lewis are present on many human cells, and are also found in animals, bacteria, and even in many plants, beans, seeds and protozoa. Interestingly renal graft survival is inferior in patients lacking Lewis antigens, suggesting that Lewis antibodies may play a role in graft rejection. Le^a and Le^b are the result of additional fucose residues on the H, A, or B

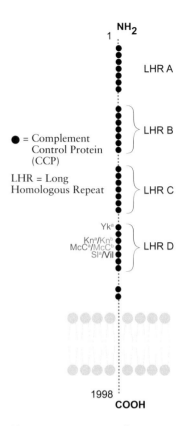

Fig. 15.31 Structure of CR1 glycoprotein (CD35)

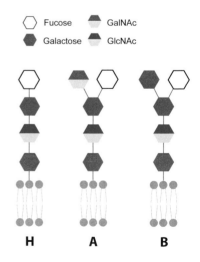

Fig. 15.33 Terminal sugars for H, A and B antigens. H is equivalent to blood group O

Table 15.3 Function, tissue distribution, and disease association for some proteins carrying blood group systems with enzyme and complement activity

Function	System name	Present in other tissue	Null Phenotype	Disease association
Enzymes				
Cleaves big endothelin 3 to ET-3, a potent vaso-constrictor	KEL	Bone marrow, fetal liver, testes, brain, lymphoid tissue, heart	K_{null} (K_0)	
Acetylcholinesterase	YT	Granulocytes, brain and muscle	1 case of congenital dyserythropoietic anemia (? acquired)	Absent from PNH III RBCs
ART4	DO	WBCs	Gy(a–)	Absent from PNH III RBCs
Complement				
Complement regulation, binds C3b; disassembles C3/C5 convertase	CROM	Vascular endothelium, GI, GU, CNS epithelia. Soluble form in plasma and urine	Inab	Absent from PNH III RBCs. Dr^a is the receptor for uropathogenic *E. coli*.
Complement regulation, binds C3b and C4b; mediates phagocytosis	KN	B lymphocytes, a subset of T lymphocytes, other nucleated blood cells, glomerular podocytes, follicular dendritic cells	Not reported	Antigens depressed in certain autoimmune and malignant conditions
Complement components	CH/RG	Plasma	C4-deficient RBCs predisposes to SLE	Certain phenotypes have increased susceptibility to certain autoimmune conditions and infections
Other				
Glycocalyx	ABO	Epithelial cells, secretions, ectoderm and endoderm	Group O	Altered expression in some hematological disorders
Glycocalyx	H	Broad distribution, soluble – all fluids except CSF in secretors	Bombay (O_h)	Decreased in some tumor cells. Increased in hematopoietic stress
Glycocalyx	LE	Blood cells, gastrointestinal tract, skeletal muscle, kidney, adrenal	Le(a–b–)	Increased expression in fucosidosis. Lewis antibodies may be important in graft rejection
Glycocalyx	I	Broad tissue distribution	i, I-negative	Congenital cataracts in Asians
Glycocalyx	GLOB	Blood cells. Soluble form in cyst fluid	p	Receptor *E. coli* and Parvovirus B19

carbohydrate chains. Clinically, the ABO antigens are most important because of blood transfusion, yet their biological function is unknown.

I blood group system: An I for an eye

Individuals with the I_{null} (I–, adult i) phenotype lack the highly branched carbohydrate chain that expresses the I blood group antigen.

In the 1970s and 1980s, it was noted that Asians with this blood type develop cataracts while Caucasians generally did not. The gene encoding the I-branching sugar (IGNT) has three alternative forms of exon 1 (1A, 1B, and 1C), with common exons 2 and 3. A nucleotide change in either exon 2 or 3 silences the gene in all tissues, including lens epithelium, resulting in the I_{null} phenotype associated with congenital cataracts. In contrast, a nucleotide change in exon 1C silences the gene in red cells but not in other tissues and leads to the I_{null} phenotype without cataracts.

The I antigen is built on the backbone of the i antigen. The i antigen is a linear structure of two repeating carbohydrates (GlcNAc and Gal) attached either to lipids via linker carbohydrates, or to asparagine in the N-glycan motif (Asn-X-Ser/Thr, where 'X' is any amino acid except proline) via a mannose rich core (Fig. 15.34). The I antigen is formed when the disaccharide (GlcNAc-Gal) is added to the linear chain in the form of numerous braches. The more branches, the stronger the expression of I antigen and the weaker the expression of i antigen.

The globoside blood group system

The P (GLOB) antigen (Fig. 14.1), is the receptor for parvovirus B19, which infects erythroid progenitors and causes benign anemia in most infected people and can cause severe aplastic crisis in patients with hypoplastic anemia. P-fimbriated strains of E. coli express both P-binding and P^k-binding molecules at the tips of their hairs, which bind to P and P^k antigens through the disaccharide galactose-galactose, and may cause pyelonephritis.

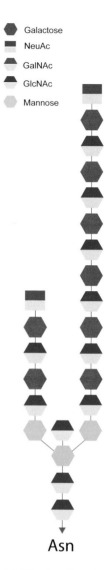

Fig. 15.34 The I antigen is expressed when the linear carbohydrate chain backbone (the i antigen) has numerous branches, consisting of repeating disaccharides

Last thought

It is often said that "Less is more". How fascinating, then, and perhaps paradoxical, that it should be the absence of a protein or a carbohydrate (as in the blood group null phenotypes) that has provided the richest source of our understanding of the activities on the surfaces of all our cells. It has also provided a spectacle that is as beautiful as the microscopic animalcules on the surface of duckweed discovered in the ditches of Delft 300 years ago. Whereas van Leeuwenhoek's Protista have had no impact on science or medicine, the structures shown above—four orders of magnitude smaller—are the keys to life.

Glossary

A

Acanthocyte An abnormally shaped red cell with a few irregular spicules.

Acetyl galactosamine An acetylated six–ring amino-sugar widely distributed in nature. Attached to the terminal sugar it forms the A antigen.

Agglutinate To clump, to cause red cells to stick together. From Latin, *ad*, to; *gluten*, glue.

Agglutination The aggregating or clumping of cells, typically by an antibody. Ottenberg commented in 1908:

> The reaction of agglutination is so striking as to lead to the thought that agglutination might be a danger in transfusion . . . it might account for some of the unfavorable results in transfusion.

AIHA see: Autoimmune hemolytic anemia

Albumin Water soluble proteins that occur in serum, milk, eggs and many tissues. Derived from the name for the white of an egg. From Latin *albus*, white.

Alkaptonuria An autosomal recessive inability to metabolize homogentisic acid which is deposited in cartilages causing early onset arthritis. It accumulates in the blood and in urine which turns dark on adding alkali, or on standing. From Arabic *al,* the; and *qali*, ashes—especially the ashes of the saltwort plant, which are alkaline.

Allele From Greek *allelon*, of one another. An allele is an alternative form of a pair or a series of genes at the same locus.

Alloantibody, synonym: **isoantibody** An antibody in the same species.

Amniotic fluid Soon after fertilization, amniotic fluid forms around the embryo, and throughout pregnancy provides an aquatic existence bounded by an amniotic sac.

Amorph A gene that is silent, NULL, it produces no detectable effect.

Antibody An immunoglobulin produced by B lymphocytes (white cells made in bone marrow). Antibodies bind to antigens and foreign molecules to inactivate them or mark them for destruction.

Anticoagulant A substance that stops blood from clotting. There are two types; indirect slow acting coumadin and indandione, and direct fast acting heparin and ancrod. Coumadin is derived from coumarin which is present in many plants, it gives new mown grass its pleasant smell.

Antigen An antigen is a cell surface marker, either a sugar or protein that is capable of stimulating the production of an antibody.

Anti-species antibodies Antibodies common to entire species that are active against other species, the strength of reaction varying directly with their phylogenetic distance.

Antithetical Refers to alternative forms of an antigen, produced by alleles e.g. E and e; K and k.

Autosome Any chromosome other than a sex chromosome. From Greek, *autos*, self; *soma*, body.

Autoimmune hemolytic anemia A hemolytic anemia due to antibodies arising against membrane glycoproteins or the patient's own red cells; usually against P or one of the Rh antigens.

B

BCAM Basal cell adhesion molecule.

BFU-E Burst forming unit-erythroid.

Bilirubin When the red cell is lysed, hemoglobin is released, and the globin is split off leaving heme—a four pyrrole ring—which is then opened to form a four-pyrrole chain called bilirubin. Chlorophyll is similar to heme, with a magnesium atom in the middle instead of iron.

Blocking antibody, synonym: **incomplete antibody.** An antibody that attaches to an antigen but cannot be demonstrated by direct agglutination.

Blood group, synonym: **blood type.** Immunologically distinct class of blood distinguished by presence or absence of antigens.

Blood Group Collections A collection is a set of antigens that are biochemically or genetically related yet with their genetics unresolved. In 2010, there were 8 Collections.

Blood Group System The ISBT defines a Blood Group System as one controlled at a single locus or by very closely linked genes.

C

CAM see: Cell adhesion molecule.

Cannula A thin tube for inserting into the body. From the diminutive of the Latin *canna*, reed.

CFU-E Colony-forming unit-erythroid.

Cell adhesion molecules (CAM) Protein on the surface of a cell that binds one cell to another or to the matrix.

Centromere A constriction in a chromosome that separates the short (p) arm from the long (q) arm.

Cesarean or C section "Macduff was from his mother's womb untimely ripped." In AD 70, Pliny the Elder (and the unreliable) said an ancestor of Caesar was delivered thus. Because maternal mortality is lower in vaginal deliveries, the World Health Organization recommends that C sections should never exceed 15% of births. Currently: in China, 46% of deliveries are by C section, in the USA, 32% and in the UK, 24%.

Chaperone A protein that helps other proteins to fold correctly and be inserted in the membrane.

Chemokine A small protein—a cellular pheromone—that attracts cells.

Chromosome An extremely long DNA molecule that carries the genes. From Greek *chroma*, color; *soma*, body, because a chromosome absorbs aniline dyes making them visible. Humans have 22 pairs of autosomes and two heterosomes, the X and Y chromosomes.

Complement A heat-stable system of serum proteins that takes part in host defense by causing lysis or phagocytosis.

Congenital idiopathic anemia A severe and progressive reduction of hemoglobin soon after birth, now known as a manifestation of HDN.

Crossing over The exchange of DNA between paired homologous chromosomes in meiosis. The visible concomitant of recombination.

Cytokine see: Chemokine.

D

DAF Decay-accelerating factor.

DARC Duffy antigen receptor for chemokines.

Disulfide bonds Thiol or sulfhydryl groups (—SH) readily form a covalent S—S bridge with another (—SH), which contributes to the 3-dimensional shape (conformation) of a protein.

Dominant The allele that is expressed phenotypically in the heterozygote. Mendel's first cross between tall and short peas gave offspring that were all tall, some being homozygous, but some tall carried a recessive allele, as in the next generation cross, 25% were short homozygous recessives.

E

Eclampsia Convulsive fits and coma during late pregnancy causing death if untreated. The cause is unknown, but it is preventable by controlling pre-eclamptic toxemia.

EDTA A crystalline acid, ethylenediamine-tetraacetic acid, which efficiently removes calcium and magnesium that is a required co-factor in clotting.

Electrophoresis The movement of charged particles, or molecules, often proteins, in a gel by means of an electric current. From Latin *electrum*, amber (the ancient Greeks rubbed amber to create electricity); and Greek *phoresis*, carrying.

Elute or **elution** Process of removing antibodies that are attached to red cells. From Latin *elutis*, washed out.

Endothelium The layer of cells that lines the blood vessels, the heart and body cavities.

Elliptocyte Elliptical shaped red cells, erroneously called ovalocytes.

Erythroblast A young, or precursor, nucleated red cell. From Greek *erythros*, red; *blastos*, germ.

Erythroblastosis The presence of erythroblasts in circulation.

Erythroblastosis fetalis Erstwhile term for HDN, with rapid red cell production both in sites that are normal (bone marrow) and ectopic (liver and spleen).

Euchromatin and heterochromatin These terms were coined by Emil Hertz in 1928 when he discovered the technique of tissue squashing that enabled him to reveal chromosomes to have dense gene-poor (heterochromatin) regions and light-staining gene-rich (euchromatin) regions.

Eugenics The study of "improving" the human race through breeding. Greek *eu,* good; *genos,* race.

Exchange transfusion Replacing the patient's blood with donated blood.

Express Cause the appearance of a gene product or an observable phenotype.

Extracellular matrix Complex network of polysaccharides and proteins secreted by cells serving as scaffolding.

F

Familial telangiectasia Dilations of the small blood vessels due to abnormal junctures of small arteries and veins. When they occur on the skin surface they appear as small red marks, when they occur in internal organs, lung, brain, or nose, they come to light when they bleed.

Fetus An unborn child between eight weeks and delivery; before that, it is an embryo.

Fibrin The white protein that forms the essential part of a blood clot.

Fimbriated Meaning fringed, from Latin *fimbriae,* fringe.

Fucose A six-carbon sugar found in seaweed that is the terminal sugar on the O/H antigen of red cells.

G

Galactose A six-carbon sugar that forms the B antigen on red cells. It combines with glucose to form lactose in the milk of all mammals except the sea lion. From Greek *galaktos,* milk.

Gamma Globulin Gamma globulins are globular shaped proteins that are antibodies against many infections and many blood group antigens.

Gene An inherited unit of the genetic code (a linear sequence of nucleotides) that is the blueprint for a specific property of a cell. Each gene has a defined location

153

on a chromosome. From Greek *genos*, race, the term gene was coined by Wilhelm Johannsen in 1909.

Genotype The overall genetic makeup of an animal or plant or more specifically the makeup at a particular locus that is responsible for a blood group antigen.

Genetics The study of the biological basis of inheritance, variation and speciation.

GPI Glycosylphosphatidylinositol.

Globin Globins are heme-containing proteins involved in oxygen binding and transport, widespread though not ubiquitous throughout the living kingdoms.

Globoside Specific sugar residues attached to lipid.

Glycoprotein A protein containing at least one carbohydrate group.

Glycerol, synonym: glycerine $C_3H_5(OH)_3$, a small organic compound, a building block of triglycerides and many proteins.

H

HDN see: Hemolytic disease of the newborn.

Helicobacter pylori A species of bacteria whose preferred residence is the human stomach, an environment that is not pleasing for any other species.

Hematopoiesis The process of making blood cells.

Heme see: Bilirubin.

Hemoglobin Hemoglobin is the major constituent of the red cell; it gives it its red color, and according to the American physiologist L.H. Henderson is the second most interesting substance in the world. It carries respiratory gasses for the majority of animal species, it occurs in many moulds, yeasts and amoebae and even in the roots of the same order of plants that have ABO antibodies in their seeds.

Hemoglobinuria Hemoglobin in the urine.

Hemolysis The puncturing or destruction of the red cell membrane causing its contents to escape.

Hemolytic Disease of the Newborn (HDN) Currently known as hemolytic disease of the fetus and newborn. A disease occurring before birth or at birth, consisting of red cell destruction caused by the mother's IgG antibodies to the child's red cell antigens crossing the placenta. The consequences are anemia, jaundice, kernicterus, erythroblastosis, hydrops, and death. Which of these manifestations occur and their severity depends on the amount of IgG entering the infant's circulation and other unknown factors.

Hemophilia An X-linked recessive bleeding disease due to a deficiency of factor VIII.

Heterophile Having affinity for other antigens or antibodies from a different species. Greek *hetero*, other or different; *philein*, to love.

HLA Human leukocyte antigen.

Homologous Having a similar position, structure, or function.

Hydrops Meaning "waterlogged", an excess of water, typically visible as edema. Dropsy is an old name.

I

ICAM Inter-cellular adhesion molecule.

Icterus gravis neonatorum One manifestation of HDN. A severe jaundice of newborn, usually appearing a few hours after birth and progressing rapidly. The color is due to bilirubin. Whenever the level of bilirubin in the blood rises above 20 milligrams/100 ml (ten times normal) it is diffusely and symmetrically deposited in the brain causing kernicterus.

IgG Abbreviation for immunoglobulin G, one of the five types of immunoglobulin found in the higher vertebrates. They are the most abundant class of immunoglobulins, they are active against Rh antigen, fungi, viruses and bacteria. The molecule is small enough to cross the placenta. (150 kilodaltons, or 7S (Svedberg units).

IgM Abbreviation for immunoglobulin M which is the first type of antibody made by the developing B lymphocyte, and it is the major type secreted into the blood on the first exposure to an antigen. The molecular weight is almost one million (19 S units), too large to pass through the placenta.

IgSF Immunoglobulin superfamily of cell surface proteins that enable cells to adhere, bind and recognize other cells.

IL Interleukins, when first described were proteins secreted by leukocytes that communicate with other leukocytes. They now are known to be widely produced in the body.

Immunoglobulin see: "antibody", "IgG", and "IgM".

Immune response The response made by the body to an invading substance.

Immunization The process of inducing immunity. Once the immune system is primed by exposure to an antigen, it will respond on subsequent challenges with enough antibodies to destroy the foreign substance.

Incomplete antibody see: blocking antibody.

Inheritance The process of genetic transmission from parents to their offspring. In 1908, Ottenberg noted:

> In one [family] the mother and seven children were all found to belong to group 2 . . . in another family, mother, father and four children all belonged to group 3. It seemed probably a coincidence that the father and mother were of the same group, but possibly a matter of heredity that the children were.

Intragroup transfusion reaction A transfusion reaction occurring when the donor and recipient are the same blood group.

Intraperitoneally Within the peritoneal cavity in the abdomen.

Intravascularly Within a blood vessel; usually a vein.

ISBT International Society of Blood Transfusion

Isoimmunization Immunization by antigens of the same species.

In vitro From Latin *vitrum*, glass, hence: in the glass test tube.

In vivo From Latin *vivere*, to live, hence: in life.

J

Jaundice From French *jaunice*, yellowness. The French drink much alcohol that damages the liver that can not excrete enough bile so it stains the eyes, skin and brain yellow. Even a normal liver can be overwhelmed if bilirubin production is excessive due to increased red cell destruction.

K

Kernicterus Brain damage due to bilirubin deposition in the brain causing cerebral palsy or deafness.

L

LAD Leukocyte adhesion deficiency.

Lectins Lectins are specific sugar binding proteins that occur in high concentration in the bean juice of the Leguminosae, and in invertebrates, compensating for lack of immune systems. They can be used to agglutinate red cells or other cells. In 1978 the Soviets killed Georgi Markov by agglutinating his red cells by shooting a pellet of castor bean lectins into his leg as he walked across Westminster bridge.

Ligand A molecule or substance that binds specifically and reversably to a site typically on a protein. From Latin *ligare*, to bind.

Locus From Latin *locus*, place, precise place of a gene on a chromosome.

Leukocytes Leukocytes defend the body against infection and foreign matter.

Lymphocyte A white blood cell with a large nucleus, one class of which produces antibodies.

Lyonization The random inactivation of one or other of the X chromosomes early in embryogenesis. It explains why two Xs are only a little better than one, not twice as good, as would be expected. (See: Mary Lyon in chapter 9).

M

Malaria A disease that infects about 250 million people a year, and kills about one million. The disease was noted to occur in the bad air, *mal ária*, of swampy land before it was realized that mosquitoes liked stagnant water for breeding and before the five species of *Plasmodium* were discovered in the gut of the female *Anopheles* mosquito. William Blake might have asked of the mosquito, as he did of the tiger:

> Did He smile His work to see?
> Did He who made the lamb make thee?

Meiosis Cell divisions that occur twice while the chromosomes replicate once thereby halving the number of chromosomes in the four descendants.

Mendelian inheritance see: Dominant.

Merozoites The name for the malarial parasite at the stage when it attacks the red cells.

Metastasis The transfer of disease, often cancer, from one part of the body to another.

Microorganism   A general term for bacteria, rickettsia, viruses, yeasts or moulds.

Monoclonal antibodies   A cell line from a hybrid of myeloma cells and antibody-secreting B cells will produce monoclonal antibody molecules that show no variation, whereas polyclonal antibodies are created naturally by many different B cells reacting with overlapping epitopes within an antigenic determinant.

N

Natural antibodies   Antibodies like anti-A or anti-B were considered natural or innate because they were always present without any stimulation. In 1959 it was discovered that they had been stimulated but the name stuck.

Natural knockouts   The null phenotypes in which there is no gene product are a naturally occurring counterpart to knockout mice that are genetically engineered to remove or inactivate a gene.

Natural selection   Nature's culling process allowing the fittest, the best adapted or the most fertile to survive. E.B. Ford and R.A. Fisher believed that natural selection would explain the observed variation in blood groups. The film of birds in Wytham Woods picking off the more visible white rather than the camouflaged black peppered moths was the first live demonstration of natural selection. It brought tears to the eyes of many zoologists.

Normocyte   The mature form of a red cell, which in most vertebrates is nucleated. In all mammals it is anucleated and in humans it also has a biconcave disc shape.

Nucleotide   A phosphorylated nucleoside. A nucleoside is a sugar linked to a purine or pyrimidine base.

O

Ovalocyte see: Elliptocyte.

P

PCH   Paroxysmal cold hemoglobinuria.

Phagocytosis   The process whereby certain white cells ingest cell debris, bacteria and any foreign bodies.

Phenotype   The characteristics of a person or organism that can be appraised biochemically or objectively measured such as baldness or blood group B.

Placenta The placenta appeared 80 million years ago as an organ to sustain the child in the uterus. In humans it is about seven inches in diameter, one inch thick. The ancient Romans called it *placenta* from Latin, a flat cake, made with cheese, a prototype pizza.

Plasma The watery supernatant of anti-coagulated blood.

Plasmapheresis The process of taking blood, removing the plasma and returning the remaining blood to the patient or donor.

Plasmodium falciparum see: malaria.

PNH Paroxysmal nocturnal hemoglobinuria.

Polyagglutination Agglutination of red cells by plasma from the majority of adults. From Greek *poly*, many.

Polymerase chain reaction (PCR) An amazing technique for amplifying a billion-fold a specific part of DNA in vitro by separating the DNA into strands, which then make copies of themselves.

Pre-eclamptic toxemia A disease of unknown cause that shows itself in the second half of pregnancy as high blood pressure, albumin in the urine and dropsy.

Proband The individual who is independently identified as affected.

Pseudoautosomal Regions of the sex chromosomes that exchange DNA as if they were on autosomes.

R

Recessive The allele that is not expressed when the dominant allele is present; this was the case with Mendel's first hybrid generation of crossed short and tall peas, none of which were short.

S

SDS Sodium dodecyl sulfate.

Sensitized Red cells to which immunoglobulins are attached.

Serum The clear fluid part of blood after it has clotted. The fibrinogen and the other clotting factors are removed, otherwise it is the same as plasma.

Sex-linkage The association of a characteristic with gender, attributed to a gene located on a sex chromosome.

Sickle cells In 1910, James Herrick and Ernest Irons found sickle shaped red cells in a dental student from the West Indies whose disease, sickle cell anemia, was soon to be described. In 1949, Linus Pauling demonstrated that these patients had red cells containing a hemoglobin that differed electrophoretically from normal.

SNP Single-nucleotide polymorphism.

Specificity A characteristic of an antibody that allows it to attach to a specific or precise antigen.

Supergene family A group of linked genes that are functionally related. The term was coined by the German botanist A. Ernst in 1936, four years after the invention of Superman.

Systemic lupus erythematosus An autoimmune collagen vascular disease typically affecting young women.

T

Thalidomide A tasteless synthetic sedative and anti-emetic that if taken in pregnancy between 37th and 54th day from the first day of the last menstrual period, caused multiple organ malformations in the fetus in about one percent of women.

Titer The concentration of a substance, usually an antibody, in solution.

Transfuse Literally, the "pouring" of blood from a bag into a person. From Latin, *trans*, across; and *fundere*, to pour.

Transfusion reaction This may include immediate or delayed hemolysis; an allergic response with urticaria, fever and bronchospasm, or there may be non-immune hazards such as heart failure and local inflammation.

U

Umbilical vein The vein that links a fetus to the placenta.

V

Virus An infectious nucleic acid-protein complex (either DNA or RNA) that replicates inside an intact host cell, usually causing disease. Landsteiner discovered that poliomyelitis was due to a filterable virus. About 5,000 types have been described.

They are abundant and ubiquitous and small enough to infect bacteria. There are 100 million times more bacteria in the ocean than stars in the known universe, and there are a thousand times more viruses than bacteria. Most of the biomass in the ocean is made up of 4×10^{30} viruses.

Sources of Information and Notes

The following Star Bright Books' modification of the Vancouver Convention—
all titles in italics, and spaces as well as punctuation are placed between numbers.
Journal titles are abbreviated as in National Library of Medicine Catalog.

CHAPTER 1 IN THE BEGINNING WAS THE ABC, PP. 3–10

Bearn AG, Miller ED. *Archibald Garrod and the development of the concept of inborn errors of metabolism.* Bull Hist Med. 1979; 53: 315.

Bordet J. *Agglutination et dissolution des globules rouges par le serum: deuxième mémoire.* Ann de l'Inst Pasteur. 1899; 13: 273.

Committee of the American Association of Immunologists. *New designations for blood groups according to iso-agglutinins.* JAMA. 1927; 88: 1421.

Creite A. *Versuche über die Wirkung des Serumeiweisses nach Injection in das Blut. Zeitschrift für Rationelle Medicin. 1869; 36: 90* (cited in Hughes-Jones NC, Gardner B. *Red cell agglutination: the first description by Creite (1869) and further observations made by Landois (1875) and Landsteiner (1901).* Br J Haematol. 2002; 119: 889-93). [Nevin Hughes-Jones unearthed and preserved Creite's contribution.]

von DeCastello A, Sturli A. *Über die Isoagglutinie im Serum gestunder und kranker Menschen.* Munch Med Wochenschr. 1902; 26: 1090.

von Dungern E, Hirszfeld L. *Concerning heredity of group specific structures of blood* (translation of *Über Vererbung gruppenspezifischer Strukturen des Blutes,II*). Z f. Immunitätsf. 1910; 6: 284—in Transfusion. 1962; 2: 70.

Dupont M. *Contribution a l'étude des antigens des globules rouges.* Arch Intern Med Exp. 1934; 9: 133.

Epstein AA, Ottenberg R. *Simple method of performing serum reactions.* Proc NY Path Soc. 1908; 8: 117.

Ehrlich P. *Wertbemessung des Diphtherieheilserums, und derentheoretische Grundlagen.* Klin Jahrb.1897; 6: 299. (Ehrlich wrote that "the first, [toxin] fitting the second [antibody] easily, as a key does a lock, to quote Emil Fischer's well known simile.")

Flexner S, Lewis PA. *Experimental epidemic poliomyelitis in monkeys.* JAMA. 1910; 22: 1780.

Gottlieb AM. *Karl Landsteiner, the melancholy genius: his time and his colleagues, 1868-1943.* Transfus Med Rev. 1998; 12: 18.

von Gruber M, Durham HE. *Eine neue Method zur raschen Erkennung des Choler-avibrios und des Typhusbacillus.* Munch Med Wochenschr. insert 1896; 43: 285.

Harris H. *Garrod's Inborn Errors of Metabolism.* London: Oxford University Press; 1963.

Hektoen L. *Isoagglutination of human corpuscles with respect to demonstration of opsonic index and to transfusion of blood.* JAMA. 1907; 48: 1739.

Janský J. *Háematologické studie u psychotik. [Hematological studies of psychotics].* Sborník klinicky; časopis pro pěstováni vědy lékařské. Archives bohèmes de médecine clinique. 1907; 85.

Kennedy JA. *Isohemagglutination: the work of Jan Janský with a critical analysis.* J Immunol. 1931; 20: 117.

Landois L. *Die Transfusion des Blutes, Leipzig: Vogel FCW; 1875* (cited in Hughes-Jones NC, Gardner B. Br J Haematol. 2002; 119: 889-93.)

Landsteiner K. *Über Agglutinationserscheinungen normalen menschlichen Blutes. [Agglutination phenomena in normal human blood.]* Wien Klin Wochenschr. 1901; 14: 1132. (English translation by Kappus AL in Transfusion. 1961; 1: 5).

Landsteiner's biography by Mackenzie GM, unpublished and incomplete at American Philosophical Society Library, Philadelphia, PA.

Landsteiner K. *Zur Kenntnis der antifermentativen, lytischen und agglutinietenden Wirkungen des Blutserums und der Lymphe.* Zentralbl Bakteriol. 1900; 27: 357.

Moss WL. *Studies on isoagglutinins and isohemolysins.* Bull Johns Hopkins Hosp. 1910; 221: 63.

Olby RC. *Origins of Mendelism.* New York: Schocken Books; 1966.

Springer GF, Horton RE, Forbes M. *Origin of anti-human blood group B agglutinins in white Leghorn chicks.* J Exp Med. 1959; 110: 221.

Widal F. *Serodiagnostic del la fievre typhoide.* Bull Soc Med Hop. 1896; 13: 561.

CHAPTER 2 BEFORE THE BEGINNING PP. 11–20

Osler W. *The Growth of Truth as Illustrated in the Discovery of the Circulation of the Blood*: Harveian lecture Royal College Physicians, London. Oct 18, 1906 in William Osler's collected papers on the Cardiovascular System, Birmingham: The Classics of Cardiology Library; 1985. p.877. Osler made a few main points, he declared that Harvey changed all of medicine (but had no influence on its current practice) by demonstrating the power of experiment, which henceforth became the source of truth, not the sages. He showed that truth is widely resisted, quoting Locke: "Truth scare ever yet carried it by vote anywhere at its first appearance." He reported the clues that lead to his discovery and he gave the lineage of hesitancy, even from the greatest, in revealing their findings. Most eureka moments are put on ice according to Osler:

> Boyle states that in the only conversation he ever had with him, Harvey acknowledged that the study of the valves of the veins had led him to the discovery of the circulation of the blood.

> Copernicus so dreaded the prejudices of mankind that he delayed publication for 30 years. Harvey delayed publication for 12 years. Between the rough sketch in 1842 and the publication of *The Origin of Species*, 17 years elapsed, and from the date of Darwin's first journal notes in 1836, more than 20 years. Napier spent nearly 20 years developing his theory of logarithms. Bacon kept *Novum Organum* by him for 12 years and year by year touched it up. Isaac Newton grasped the secret of cosmic circulation in silence for more than 20 years before publishing *Principia*.

Pepys S. *The diary of Samuel Pepys*. Robert Latham and William Matthews editors, Berkeley and LA: University of California Press; 1972. vii. p.370.

Russell B. *A history of western philosophy*. New York: Simon and Schuster; 1945.

Stansbury LG, Hess JR. *Blood transfusion in World War I: The roles of Lawrence Bruce Robertson and Oswald Hope Robertson in the "most important medical advance of the war"*. Transfus Med Rev. 2009; 23: 232.

Weatherall D J. *Haematology in the new millennium*. Brit J Haematol. 2000; 108: 1.

Chapter 3 In Search of Other Blood Groups, pp. 21-26

Chalmers JNM, Ikin EW, Mourant AE. *A study of two unusual blood-group antigens in West Africans*. Br Med J. 1953; ii: 175.

Landsteiner K. *The specificity of serological reactions*. Cambridge: Harvard University Press; 1946.

Landsteiner K, Levine P. *A new agglutinable factor differentiating individual human bloods*. Proc Soc Exp Biol Med. 1927; 24: 600.

Landsteiner K, Levine P. *Further observations on individual differences of human blood*. Proc Soc Exp Biol Med. 1927; 24: 941.

Landsteiner K, Levine P. *On the inheritance of agglutinogens of human blood demonstrable by immune agglutinins*. J Exp Med. 1928; 48: 731.

Landsteiner K, Levine P. *On individual differences in human blood*. J Exp Med. 1928; 47: 757.

Landsteiner K, Levine P. *Experiments on anaphylaxis to azoproteins: Third Paper*. J Exp Med. 1930; 52: 347.

Landseiner K, Strutton WR, Chase M. *An agglutination reaction observed with some human bloods, chiefly among negroes*. J Immunol. 1934; 27: 469.

Levine P. *A review of Landsteiner's contributions to human blood groups. Transfusion.* 1961; 1: 45.

Mazumdar PMH. *Species and specificity: an interpretation of the history of immunology.* Cambridge: Cambridge University Press; 1995.

CHAPTER 4 RUTH DARROW'S INSIGHT, PP. 27–32

Buhrman WL, Sanford HN. *Is familial jaundice of newborn infants erythroblastosis fetalis?* Am J Dis Child. 1931; 41: 225.

Damashek W, Greenwalt TJ, Tat RJ. *Erythroblastosis fetalis (acute hemolytic anemia of the newborn.* Am J Dis Child. 1943; 65: 571.

Darrow RR. *Icterus gravis (erythroblastosis) neonatorum: an examination of etiologic considerations.* Arch Pathol. 1938; 25: 378.

Diamond LK, Blackfan KD, Baty JM. *Erythroblastosis fetalis and its association with universal edema of the fetus, icterus gravis neonatorum and anemia of the newborn.* J Pediatr. 1932; 1: 269.

Dienst A. Das *Eklampsiegift.* Zentralbl Gynakol. 1905; 12: 353.

Ferguson JA. *Erythroblastosis with jaundice and edema in the newly born.* Am J Pathol. 1931; 7: 277.

Halban J. *Agglutinationsversuche mit muuterlichen und kinderlichen blute.* Wien Klin Wochenschr. 1900; 13: 545. [He suggested isoimmunization causes haemoblastosis.]

Levine P. *Historical perspectives before 1945.* Typescript of 1980 book chapter, probably for 11th Annual Scientific Symposium. American Red Cross, 1979. *Immunobiology of the erythrocyte.* In Ottenberg archives, Mt Sinai Hospital NY.

McQuarrie I. *Isoagglutination in new-born infants and their mothers, a possible relationship between interagglutination and the toxemias of pregnancy.* Bull Johns Hopkins Hosp. 1923; 34: 51.

Ottenberg R. *The etiology of eclampsia.* JAMA. 1923; 81: 4, 295.

Panaroli D. *Iatrologismorum sive observationum medicinalium.* Pentacostae quarta. obs. 1654; 44: 137.

Wiener AS. *Diagnosis and treatment of anemia of the newborn caused by occult placental hemorrhage.* Am J Obstet Gynecol. 1948; 56: 717.

Zuelzer WW. *Pediatric Hematology in Historical Perspective.* In: Nathan DG, Orski FA, editors. *Hematology of Infancy and Childhood.* 3rd ed. Philadelphia: WB Saunders Co. 1987. p.10.

Chapter 5 Discovery of Rh, pp. 33–38

Chown B. *Never transfuse a woman with her husband's blood.* CMAJ. 1949; 61: 419.

Levine P, Stetson R. *An unusual case of intra-group agglutination.* JAMA. 1939; 113: 126. (also in JAMA 1984; 251: 1316).

Levine P, Vogel P, Katzin EM, Burnham L. *Pathogenesis of erythroblastosis fetalis: statistical evidence.* Science. 1941; 94: 371.

Levine P, Katzin EM, Burnham L. *Isoimmunization in pregnancy. Its possible bearing on the etiology of erythroblastosis foetalis.* JAMA. 1941; 116: 825.

Levine P, Burnham L, Katzin EM, Vogel P. *The role of iso-immunization in the pathogenesis of erythroblastosis fetalis.* Am J Obstet Gynecol. 1941; 42: 925.

Reid ME. Alexander S. Wiener: *The man and his work.* Transfus Med Rev. 2008; 22: 300.

Rosenfield RE. *Early twentieth century origins of modern blood transfusion therapy.* Mt Sinai J Med. 1974; 41: 626.

Stetson RE. *Causes and prevention of posttransfusion reactions.* Surg Clin North Am. 1933; 13: 319.

Wiener AS. *Diagnosis and treatment of anemia of the newborn caused by occult placental hemorrhage.* Am J Obstet Gynecol. 1948; 56: 717.

Chapter 6 Rh HDN: Treatment & Prevention, pp. 39–56

Bevis DCA. *Antenatal Prediction of Haemolytic Disease of the Newborn.* Lancet. 1952; i: 395.

Chown B. *Anemia from bleeding of the fetus into the mother's circulation.* Lancet. 1954; i: 1213.

Chown B. *The fetus can bleed: three clinico-pathological pictures.* Am J Obstet Gynecol. 1955; 70: 1298.

Clarke CA, Finn R, McConnell RB, Sheppard PM. *The protection afforded by ABO incompatability against erythroblastosis due to Rhesus anti-D.* Int Arch Allergy Immunol. 1958; 13: 377.

Clarke CA, Donohoe WTA, McConnell RB, Finn R, Krevans JR, Kulke W, Lehane D, Sheppard PM. *Further experimental studies on the prevention of Rh haemolytic disease.* Br Med J. 1963; 1: 979.

Clarke CA, Finn R. *Prevention of Rh hemolytic disease: background of the Liverpool work.* Am J Obstet Gynecol. 1977; 127(5): 538.

Cremer RJ, Perryman PW, Richards DH. *Influence of light on the hyperbilirubinaemia of infants.* Lancet. 1958; 271: 1094.

Discovery and Significance of Blood Groups

Cross, GK. *Report on blood transfusion work seen in the Hospital for Sick Children, Toronto, Canada.* British Journal of Children's Diseases. 1924; 21: 173.

Darrow RR. *The treatment of erythroblastosis fetalis.* JAMA. 1945; 127: 1146.

Diamond LK. *Erythroblastosis foetalis or haemolytic disease of the newborn.* Proc R Soc Med. 1947; 40: 546.

Diamond, LK. *Erythroblastosis fetalis treated by replacement transfusion via the umbilical vein.* Am J Dis Child. 1948; 75: 457.

Dienst A. Das Eklampsiegift. Zentralbl Gynakol 1905; 12: 353.

Doppler. *ACOG Practice Bulletin No. 75: Management of alloimmunization.* Obstet Gynecol. 2006; 108: 457.

Finn R. Typescripts of talks with similar titles and similar themes:

Erythroblastosis. Medical Institution, [Liverpool 1960].

The Protective mechanisms against erythroblastosis. Liverpool University Medical Sciences Club, 22 Feb. 1960; reported in summary: Erythroblastosis. 1960. Lancet; i: 526.

The Protective factors in erythroblastosis. 1960; 133rd meeting British Genetical Society, typescript in archives at University of Wyoming.

Protective mechanisms against erythroblastosis. Typescript of talk to Association of Physicians, April 1961. This talk concludes:

> the injection of anti-D into the mother should either destroy or inactivate these cells and thus prevent the subsequent occurrence of haemolytic disease in a future pregnancy.

Protective mechanisms against erythroblastosis. 2nd International Congress of Human Genetics, Sept. 1961.

Peripatetic Club, Boston, Feb 1962.

Columbia University Seminar, May 1962.

Mt Sinai Obs-Gyn conference, April 1962.

Finn R. *Protective mechanisms against Rh haemolytic disease.* MD [dissertation]. Liverpool, England: University of Liverpool; 1961.

Flexner S. *On Thrombi composed of agglutinated red blood corpuscles.* Journal of Medical Research. 1902; 8(2): 316.

Freda VJ, Gorman JG, Pollack W. *Prevention of Rh-hemolytic disease with Rh-immune globulin.* Am J Obstet Gynecol. 1977; 128: 456.

Freda VJ, Gorman JG, Pollack W, Bowe E. *Prevention of Rh hemolytic disease--ten years' clinical experience with Rh immune globulin.* N Engl J Med. 1975; 292: 1014.

168

Freda V. *Hemolytic disease*. Clin Obstet Gynecol. 1973; 1: 72.

Gladstone G, Abraham EP. *Biological factors in the production of antibodies*. In: Howard W. Florey HW, editor. General Pathology. 2nd ed. Philadelphia: W. B. Saunders Company: 1959.

Gorman JG. *The Role of the laboratory in hemolytic disease of the newborn*. Philadelphia: Lea & Febiger; 1975. p.125.

Gorman JG. In an interview in 2004, we asked John Gorman for any documentation of his original ideas, he replied:

> In July 1960 I finished my pathology residency at Columbia and joined the department. In October 1960, Dr McKay, the new chairman, called me in to his office and asked me if there were any research projects I would like to propose as there was funding readily available for New York researchers from the Health Research Council of the City of New York. I responded with the two immunology ideas: I am sure we discussed the Rh immune suppression of Rh negative mothers inspired by the Gladstone chapter which Vince Freda and I had been talking about and that was well developed at that time. Along with the idea that tolerance was an active immune response, the competition theory. However, the first surviving Rh study document seems to be the application to the Health Research Council submitted in Feb 61.

Hamilton EG. *Prevention of Rh isoimmunization by injection of anti-D antibody*. Obstet Gynecol. 1967; 6: 812.

Hamilton EG. *Ten-year experience with high titer anti-D plasma for the prevention of Rh isoimmunization*. Obstet Gynecol. 1972; 40: 692.

Hart AP. *Familial icterus gravis of the newborn and its treatment*. CMAJ. 1925; 15: 1008.

Hirszfeld L, Zborowski H. *Relationship between mother and fetus and elective permeability of the placenta on the bases of the serological coexistence between mother and fetus*. Klin Wochenschr. 1925; 24: 1152.

Hirszfeld L. Zborowski H. *Fundamentals of serologic symbiosis between mother and fetus*. Klin Wochenschr. 1926; 17: 741.

Hughes-Jones NC. *The estimation of the concentration and equilibrium constant anti-D*. Immunology. 1967; 12: 565.

Kleihauer E, Braun H, Betke K. *Demonstration of foetal hemoglobin erythrocytes by elution*. Klin Wochenschr. 1975; 35: 637.

Levine P, Vogel P, Katzin EM, Burnham L. *Pathenogenesis of erythroblastosis fetalis; statistical evidence*. Science. 1941; 94: 371.

Levine P. *Serological factors as possible causes in spontaneous abortion*. J Hered. 1943; 34 : 71.

Lewis M. Chown B. *Hidden anti-Rhesus saline antibodies*. Nature. 1954; 173: 44.

Lo YMD, Corbetta N, Chamberlain PF, Rai V, Sargent IL, Redman CWG, Wainscoat JS. *Presence of fetal DNA in maternal plasma and serum*. Lancet. 1997; 350: 485.

Loutit JF, Mollison PL, Young IM, Lucas EJ. *Citric acid-sodium citrate-glucose mixture for blood storage*. Q J Exp Physiol. 1943; 32: 183.

McQuarrie I. 1923. ibid. chapter 4.

Mollison PL. *The survival of transfused erythrocytes in haemolytic disease of the newborn*. Arch Dis Child. 1943; 18: 161.

Mollison PL. *Blood Transfusion in Clinical Medicine*. 7th ed. Oxford: Blackwell Scientific Publications; 1983.

Mollison PL. 1983; ibid. *Optimal IgG dose to prevent immunization*. p.382.

Mollison PL. 1983; ibid. *First anti-K in a mother whose baby had HDN but without anti-D*. p.344.

Mollison PL. *The Rhesus factor and disease prevention*. 2003. p.9. Wellcome Trust for the History of Medicine, available at: http://www.neonatology.org/pdf/WellcomeVol22RhDisease.pdf

Mollison PL. *Measurement of survival and destruction of red cells in haemolytic syndromes*. Br Med Bull. 1959; 15: 59.

Orkin SH, Nathan DG, Ginsburg D, Thomas Look AT, Fisher DE, Lux S IV. *Nathan and Oski's hematology of infancy and childhood*. 7th ed. Philadelphia, PA: Saunders & Mosby; 2008.

Nevanlinna HR, Vainio T. *The Influence of Mother-Child ABO Incompatibility on Rh Immunisation*. Vox Sang. 1956; 1: 26.

Ottenberg R. 1923; ibid. chapter 4.

Thomas Paine. Thomas Paine of Thetford, England was admired by Napoleon, Jefferson, Franklin, and Washington. Paine was one of the founding fathers of the United States whose books and pamphlets were widely read, in one of which he expressed his opinions on dreams: "I pay no regard to my own dreams, and I should be weak indeed to put my faith in the dreams of another."

Race RR, Sanger R. *Blood Groups in Man*. 1950; Oxford: Blackwell Scientific Publications; 1950. p.290.

Schröder Jim. *Transplacental passage of blood cells*. J Med Genet. 1975; 12: 230.

Sidbury JB. *Transfusion through the umbilical vein in haemorrhage of the new-born*. Am J Dis Child. 1923; 25: 290.

Smith T. *Active immunity produced by so-called balanced or neutral mixtures of diphtheria toxin and antitoxin*. J Exp Med. 1909; 11: 241.

Stern K, Goodman HS, Berger M. *Experimental isoimmunisation to hemoantigens in man*. Presented at the American Association of Blood Banks in San Francisco, August 1960. J Immunol. 1961; 87: 189.

Villari, P. *La storia di Girolamo Savonarola*. Firenze, 1859, p.140.

Warrell DA, Cox TM, Firth JD, editors. *Weatherall's Oxford Textbook of Medicine*. 5th ed. Oxford, UK: Oxford Medical Publications; 2010.

Wallerstein H. *Treatment of severe erythroblastosis by simultaneous removal and replacement of the blood of the newborn infant*. Science. 1946; 103: 583.

Wiener AS, Wexler IB. *The use of heparin when performing exchange blood transfusion in new born infants*. J Lab Clin Med. 1946; 31: 1016.

Wiener AS. *Diagnosis and treatment of anemia of the newborn caused by occult placental hemorrhage*. Am J Obstet Gynecol. 1948; 56: 717.

Winbaum ES. *Immunization of Rh-negative Mother with Rh Antisera*. Pediatrics. 1968; 42: 214.

Woodrow JC. *The Rhesus factor and disease prevention*. 2003; Wellcome Trust for the History of Medicine, available at: http://www.neonatology.org/pdf/WellcomeVol22RhDisease.pdf

Woodrow JC, Finn R. *Transplacental haemorrhage*. Brit J Haematol. 1966; 12: 297.

Zimmerman D. *Rh: The intimate history of a disease and its conquest*. New York: Macmillan; 1973. He gives excellent detail of the New York meeting (p.265) as well as a fine history of the disease.

Zipursky A, Hull A, White FD, Israels FD. *Foetal erythrocytes in the maternal circulation*. Lancet. 1959; i: 451.

Zipursky A, Israels LG. *The pathogenesis and prevention of Rh immunization*. CMAJ. 1967; 97: 1245.

Chapter 7 More Antigens Revealed, pp. 57–60

Callender ST, Race RR. *A serological and genetical study of multiple antibodies formed in response to blood transfusion by a patient with lupus erythematosus diffusus*. Ann Eugen. 1946; 13: 102.

Landsteiner K, Wiener AS. *Studies on an agglutinogen (Rh) in human blood reacting with anti-rhesus sera with human isoantibodies*. J Exp Med. 1941; 74: 309.

Race RR. *An "incomplete" antibody in human serum*. Nature. 1944; 153: 771.

Sneath JS, Sneath PHA. *Adsorption of blood-group substances from serum on to red cells*. Br Med Bull. 1959; 15: 154.

Chapter 8 The Coombs Revolution, pp. 61–66

Coombs RRA. *The conglutinin and sensitization reactions*. PhD [dissertation]. Cambridge: Cambridge University; 1946.

Coombs R. Interview, 2004.

Coombs RRA, Mourant AE, Race RR. *A new test for detection of weak and incomplete agglutinins.* Br J Exp Path. 1945; 26: 255.

Moreschi C. *Neue Tatsachen über die Blutkorperchen-agglutination.* Zentralbl Bakteriol. 1908; 46: 49.

Moreschi C. *Beschleunigung und Verstarkung der Bakterienagglutination durch Eiweisssera.* Zentralbl Bakteriol. 1908; 46: 456.

CHAPTER 9 MANY MORE ANTIGENS REVEALED, PP. 67–80

Allen FH, Diamond LK, Niedziela B. *A new blood-group antigen.* Nature. 1951; 167: 482.

Bodmer WF. *Early British discoveries in human genetics: contributions of R.A, Fisher and J.B.S. Haldane to the development of blood groups.* Am J Hum Genet. 1992; 50: 671.

Coombs RRA, Mourant AE, Race RR. *In-vivo isosensitization of red cells in babies with haemolytic disease.* Lancet. 1946; i: 264.

Copeland SR, Sponheimer M, de Ruiter DJ, Lee-Thorp JA, Codron D, le Roux PJ, Grimes V, Richards MP. *Strontium isotope evidence for landscape use by early hominins.* Nature. 2011; 474: 76.

Cutbush M, Mollison PL, Parkin DM. *A new human blood group.* Naure. 1950; 165: 188.

Cutbush M, Mollison PL. *The Duffy blood group system.* Heredity. 1950; 4: 383.

Fisher RA. *The design of experiments.* Edinburgh; Oliver & Boyd: 1935.

Fisher RA. *The theory of inbreeding.* Edinburgh & London; Oliver and Boyd:1965. p.4.

Goodfellow PN, Tippett P. *A human quantitative polymorphism related to Xg blood groups.* Nature. 1981; 289: 404.

van der Hart M, Szalory A, van Loghem JJ. *A "new" antibody associated with the Kell blood group system.* Vox Sang. 1968; 15: 456.

Holman CA. *A new rare human blood-group antigen (Wr^a).* Lancet. 1953; 265: 119-20.

Ikin EW, Mourant AE, Pettenkofer HJ, Blumenthal G. *Discovery of the expected haemagglutinin, anti-Fy^b.* Nature. 1951; 168: 1077.

Levine P, Backer M, Wigod M, Ponder R. *A new human hereditary blood property (cellano) present in 99.8% of all bloods.* Science. 1949; 109: 464.

Levine P, Kuhmichel AB, Wigod M, Koch E. *A new blood factor, s, allelic to S.* Proc Soc Exp Biol Med. 1951; 78: 218.

Levine P, Bobbitt O, Waller RK, Kuhmichel A. *Isoimmunization by a new blood factor in tumor cells.* Proc Soc Exp Biol Med. 1951; 77: 403.

Levine P, Stock AH, Kuhmichel AB, Bronikovsky N. *A new human blood factor of rare incidence in the general population.* Proc Soc Exp Biol Med. 1951; 77: 402.

Lyon MF. *Gene action in the X-chromosome of the mouse (Mus musculus L.).* Nature. 1961; 190: 370.

Lyon MF. *Genetic factors on the X chromosome.* Lancet. 1961; ii: 434.

Marsh WL, Redman CM. *The Kell blood group system: A review.* Transfusion. 1990; 30: 158.

Marsh WL, Redman CM. *Recent developments in the Kell blood group system.* Transfus Med Rev 1987; 1: 4.

Mourant AE. *A new Rhesus antibody.* Nature. 1945; 155; 542.

Plaut G, Ikin EW, Mourant AE, Sanger R, Race RR. *A new blood group antibody, anti Jk^b.* Nature. 1953; 171: 431.

Sanger R, Race RR. *Subdivisions of the MN blood groups in man.* Nature. 1947; 160: 505.

Sanger R, Race RR, Walsh RJ, Montgomery C. *An antibody which subdivides the human MN blood groups.* Heredity. 1948; 2: 131.

Sussman LN, Miller EB. *Un nouveau facteur s anguine "Vel".* Rev Hematol. 1952; 7: 368.

Tippett P, Ellis NA. *The Xg blood group system: A review.* Transfus Med Rev. 1998; 12: 233.

Tippett P, Reid ME, Poole J, Green CA, Daniels GL, Anstee DJ. *The Miltenberger subsystem: is it obsolescent?* Transfus Med Rev. 1992; 6: 170.

Walsh RJ, Montgomery C. *A new human isoagglutinin subdividing the MN blood groups.* Nature. 1947; 160: 504.

Wiener AS, Unger LJ, Gordon EB. *Fatal hemolytic transfusion reaction caused by sensitization to a new blood factor U.* JAMA. 1953; 153: 1444.

Wiener AS, Unger LJ, Cohen L, Feldman J. *Type-specific cold auto-antibodies as a cause of acquired hemolytic anemia and hemolytic transfusion reactions: Biologic test with bovine red cells.* Ann Intern Med. 1956; 44: 221.

Wright Sewall, interview, 1976.

Chapter 10 Blood Group Systems and Beyond, pp. 81–88

Blumenfeld OO, Adamany AM. *Structural polymorphism within the amino-terminal region of MM, NN, and MN glycoproteins (glycophorins) of the human erythrocyte membrane*. Proc Natl Acad Sci USA. 1978; 75: 2727.

Crawford MN. *The Lutheran blood group system: serology and genetics. In: Pierce SR, Macpherson CR, editors. Blood Group Systems: Duffy, Kidd and Lutheran.* Arlington: American Association of Blood Banks; 1988. p.93.

Furthmayer H. *Structural comparison of glycophorins and immunochemical analysis of genetic variants.* Nature. 1978; 271: 519.

Huang CH, Guizzo ML, McCreary J, Leigh EM, Blumenfeld OO. *Typing of MNSs blood group specific sequences in the human genome and characterization of a restriction fragment tightly linked to S–s– alleles.* Blood. 1991; 77: 381.

Huang CH, Blumenfeld OO. *MNSs blood groups and major glycophorins: Molecular basis for allelic variation. In: Cartron J-P, Rouger P, editors. Molecular basis of human blood group antigens.* New York: Plenum Press; 1995. p.153.

Lewis M, Anstee DJ, Bird GWG, Brodheim E, Cartron J-P, Contreras M, Dahr W. *Blood group terminology 1990. ISBT working party on terminology for red cell surface antigens.* Vox Sang. 1990; 58: 152.

Shows TB, Alper CA, Bootsma D, Dorf M, Douglas T, Huisman T, Kit S, Klinger HP, Kozak C, Lalley PA, Lindsley D, McAlpine PJ, et al. *International system for human gene nomenclature (1979).* Cytogenet Cell Genet. 1979; 25: 96.

Tomita M, Marchesi VT. *Amino-acid sequence and oligosaccharide attachment sites of human erythrocyte glycophorin.* Proc Natl Acad Sci USA. 1975; 72: 2964.

Tomita M, Furthmayer H, Marchesi VT. *Primary structure of human erythrocyte glycophorin A. Isolation and characterization of peptides and complete amino acid sequence.* Biochemistry. 1978; 17: 4756.

Udden MM, Umeda M, Hirano Y, Marcus DM. *New abnormalities in the morphology, cell surface receptors, and electrolyte metabolism of In(Lu) erythrocytes.* Blood. 1987; 69: 52.

CHAPTER 11 CHROMOSOMAL ASSIGNMENTS, PP.89–98

Balbiani EG. *Sur la structure du noyau des cellules salivaires chez les larves de Chironomus.* Zool. Anz. 1881: 4: 637

Bell J, Haldane JBS. *Genes for Colour-blindness and Haemophilia in Man.* Proc R Soc Lond B Biol Sci. 1937; 123: 119.

Chalmers JNM, Lawler SD. *Data on linkage in man: Elliptocytosis and blood groups.* Ann Eugen. 1953; 17: 267.

Cook PJL. *The Lutheran-secretor recombination fraction in man: A possible sex-difference.* Ann Hum Genet. 1965; 28: 393.

Donahue RP, Bias W, Renwick JH, McKusick, V. A. *Probable assignment of the Duffy blood group locus to chromosome 1 in man.* Proc Natl Acad Sci USA. 1968; 61: 949.

Giblett ER. *Genetic Markers in Human Blood.* Oxford and Edinburgh: Blackwell Scientific Publications; 1969.

Goodall HB, Hendry DWW, Lawler SD, Stephen SA. *Data on linkage in man: Elliptocytosis and blood groups.* Ann Eugen. 1953; 17: 272.

Heitz E, Bauer H. *Beweise für die Chromosomennatur der Kernschleifen in den Knäuelkernen von Bibio hortulanus I. (Cytologische Untersuchungen an Dipteren, 1).* Z. Zellforsch. Mikrosk. Anat. 1933, 17: 67

Mann JD, Cahan A, Gelb AG, Fisher N, Hamper J, Tippett P, Sanger R, Race RR. *A sex-linked blood group.* Lancet 1962; 1: 8.

Mohr J. *A search for linkage between the Lutheran blood group and other hereditary characters.* APMIS. 1951; 28: 80.

Morton NE. *The detection and estimation of linkage between the genes for elliptocytosis and the Rh blood type.* Am J Hum Genet. 1956; 8: 80.

Painter TS. *Salivary chromosomes and the attack on the gene.* J Hered. 1934; 25: 464.

Renwick JH, Schulze J. *Male and female recombination fractions for the nail-patella: ABO linkage in man.* Ann Hum Genet. 1965; 28: 379.

Sanger R, Race RR. *The Lutheran-secretor linkage in man: Support for Mohr's findings.* Heredity. 1958; 12: 513.

Tijo JH, Levan A. *The chromosome number in man.* Hereditas. 1956; 42: 1.

Wiener AS. *Blood Groups and Transfusion.* 3rd ed. Springfield, IL: Charles C. Thomas; 1943.

Zacharias H. *Emil Heitz (1892-1965): Chloroplasts, Heterochromatin and Polytene Chromosomes.* In: *Perspectives Anecdotal, Historical and Critical Commentaries on Genetics,* editors JF Crow, WF Dove. Genetics. 1995; 141: 7.

CHAPTER 12 POWER OF TECHNIQUES, PP. 99–102

Avent ND. *Large-scale blood group genotyping: clinical implications.* Br J Haematol. 2009; 144: 13.

Denomme GA, Rios M, Reid ME. *Molecular protocols in transfusion medicine.* San Diego: Academic Press; 2000.

Denomme GA, Shahcheraghi A, Blackall DP, Oza KK, Garratty G. *Inhibition of erythroid progenitor cell growth by anti-Ge3.* Br J Haematol. 2006; 133: 443.

Hashmi G, Shariff T, Zhang Y, Cristobal J, Chau C, Seul M, Vissavajjhala P, Baldwin C, Hue-Roye K, Charles-Pierre D, et al. *Determination of 24 minor red blood cell antigens for more than 2000 blood donors by high-throughput DNA analysis.* Transfusion. 2007; 47: 736.

Hillyer CD, Shaz BH, Winkler AM, Reid ME. *Integrating molecular technologies for red blood cell typing and compatibility testing into blood centers and transfusion services.* Transfus Med Rev. 2008; 22: 117.

Köhler G, Milstein C. *Continuous cultures of fused cells secreting antibody of pre-defined specificity.* Nature. 1975; 256: 495.

Lögdberg L, Reid ME, Miller JL. *Cloning and genetic characterization of blood group carrier molecules and antigens.* Transfus Med Rev. 2002; 16: 1.

Lögdberg L, Reid ME, Lamont RE, Zelinski T. *Human blood group genes. 2004: chromosomal locations and cloning strategies.* Transfus Med Rev. 2005; 19: 45.

Micieli JA, Wang D, Denomme GA. *Anti-glycophorin C induces mitrochondrial membrane depolarization and a loss of extracellular regulated kinase ½ protein kinase activity that is prevented by pretreatment with cytochalasin D: implications for hemolytic disease of the fetus and newborn caused by anti-Ge3.* Transfusion. 2010; 50: 1761.

Morgan WT. *A contribution to human biochemical genetics; the chemical basis of blood-group specificity.* Proc R Soc Lond B Biol Sci. 1960; 151: 308.

Perreault J, Lavoie J, Painchaud P, Cote M, Constanzo-Yanez J, Côté R, Delage G, Gendron F, Dubuc S, Caron B, Lemieux R, St-Louis M. *Set-up and routine use of a database of 10,555 genotyped blood donors to facilitate the screening of compatible blood components for alloimmunized patients.* Vox Sang. 2009; 97: 61.

Reid ME. *From DNA to blood groups.* Immunohematology. 2008; 24: 166.

Reid ME. *Applications and experience with PCR-based assays to predict blood group antigens.* Transfus Med Hemother. 2009; 36: 168.

Reid ME. *Milestones in laboratory procedures and techniques.* Immunohematology 2009; 25: 39.

Saiki, R., Scharf, S., Faloona, F., Mullis, K., Horn, G., and Erlich, H. *Enzymatic amplification of beta-globin genomic sequences and restriction site analysis for diagnosis of sickle cell anemia.* Science. 1985; 230: 1350.

Vaughan JI, Manning M, Warwick RM, Letsky EA, Murray NA, Roberts IAG. *Inhibition of erythroid progenitor cells by anti-Kell antibodies in fetal alloimmune anemia.* N Engl J Med. 1998; 338: 798.

Watkins WM. *Biochemistry and genetics of the ABO, Lewis, and P blood group systems.* Adv Hum Genet. 1980; 10:1.

CHAPTER 13 BLOOD GROUPS AND DISEASE, PP. 103–112

Aird I, Bentall HH, Mehigan JA, Fraser Roberts JA. *The blood groups in relation to peptic ulceration and carcinoma of colon, rectum, breast, and bronchus: bronchus; an association between the ABO groups and peptic ulceration.* Br Med J. 1954; 2: 315.

Beardmore JA, Karimi-Booshehri F. *ABO genes are differentially distributed in socioeconomic groups in England.* Nature. 1983; 303: 522.

Boren T, Falk P, Roth KA, Larson G, Normark S. *Attachment of Helicobacter pylori to human gastric epithelium mediated by blood group antigens.* Science. 1993; 262: 1892.

Cserti CM, Dzik WH. *The ABO blood group system and Plasmodium falciparum malaria.* Blood. 2007; 110:2250.

D'Adamo PJ. *Eat Right 4 Your Type.* New York: GP Putnam's Sons; 1997.

D'Adamo PJ. *Cook Right 4 Your Type.* New York: GP Putnam's Sons; 1999.

Dausset J, Moullec J, Bernard J. *Acquired hemolytic anemia with polyagglutinability of red blood cells due to a new factor present in normal human serum (anti-Tn).* Blood. 1959; 14: 1079.

Desai, PR. *Immunoreactive T and Tn antigens in malignancy: Role in carcinoma diagnosis, prognosis, and immunotherapy.* Transfus Med Rev. 2000; 14: 312.

Garratty G. *Do blood groups have a biological role?* In: Garratty G, editor. *Immunobiology of transfusion medicine.* New York (NY): Dekker; 1994. p.201.

Garratty G. *Blood groups and disease: a historical perspective.* Transfus Med Rev. 2000; 14: 291.

Gibson JR, Harrison GA, Clarke VA, Hiorns RW. *IQ and ABO blood groups.* Nature. 1973; 246: 498.

Glinsky GV, Ivanova AB, Welsh J, McClelland M. *The role of blood group antigens in malignant progression, apoptosis resistance, and metastatic behavior.* Transfus Med Rev. 2000; 114: 326.

Hakomori S. *Fucolipids and blood group glycolipids in normal and tumor tissue.* Prog Biochem Pharmacol. 1975; 10: 167.

Hakomori S. *Philip Levine Award Lecture: blood group glycolipid antigens and their modifications as human cancer antigens.* Am J Clin Pathol. 1984; 82: 635.

Hakomori S: *Aberrant glycosylation in tumors and tumor-associated carbohydrate antigens.* Adv Cancer Res. 1989; 52: 257.

Hirschberg CB. *Golgi nucleotide sugar transport and leukocyte adhesion deficiency II.* J Clin Invest. 2001; 108: 3.

Kannagi R, Levine P, Watanabe K, Hakomori S. *Recent studies of glycolipid and glycoprotein profiles and characterization of the major glycolipid antigen in gastric cancer of a patient of blood group genotype pp (Tjᵃ-) first studied in 1951.* Cancer Res. 1982; 42: 5249.

Langman MJS, Doll R. *ABO blood group and secretor status in relation to clinical characteristics of peptic ulcers.* Gut. 1965; 6: 270.

Levine P, Bobbitt OB, Waller RK, Kuhmichel A. *Isoimmunization by a new blood factor in tumor cells.* Proc Soc Exp Biol Med. 1951; 77: 403.

Levine P. *Blood group and tissue genetic markers in familial adenocarcinoma: Potential specific immunotherapy.* Semin Oncol. 1978; 5: 25.

Levine P. *Self-nonself concept for cancer and diseases previously known as "autoimmune" diseases (illegitimate transferases/plasma exchange).* Proc Natl Acad Sci USA. 1978; 75: 5697.

Luhn K, Wild MK, Eckhardt M, Gerardy-Schahn R, Vestweber D. *The gene defective in leukocyte adhesion deficiency II encodes a putative GDP-fucose transporter.* Nat Genet. 2001; 28: 69.

Merikas G, Christakopoulos P, Petropoulos E. *Distribution of ABO blood groups in patients with ulcer disease: Its relationship to gastroduodenal bleeding.* Am J Dig Dis 1966; 11: 790.

Moreau R, Dausset J, Bernard J, Moullec J. *Acquired hemolytic anemia with polyagglutinability of erythrocytes by a new factor present in normal blood.* Bull Mem Soc Med Hop Paris. 1957; 73: 569.

Moulds JM, Moulds JJ. *Blood group associations with parasites, bacteria, and viruses.* Transfus Med Rev. 2000; 14: 302.

Mourant AE, Kopec AC, Domainiewska-Sobczak K. *Blood-groups and blood-clotting.* Lancet. 1971; i: 223.

Mourant AE, Kopec AC, and Domaniewska-Sobczak K. *Blood groups and diseases: a study of associations of diseaseas with blood groups and other polymorphisms.* Oxford: Oxford University Press; 1978.

Muschel LH. *Blood groups, disease, and selection.* Bacteriol Rev. 1966; 30: 427.

Nomi T, Besher A. *You are your blood type: the biochemical key to unlocking the secrets of your personality.* New York, NY: Pocket Books; 1988.

Preston AE, Barr A: *The plasma concentration of factor VIII in the normal population. II. The effects of age, sex and blood group.* Br J Haematol. 1964; 10: 238.

Prokop O, Uhlenbruck G. *Human Blood and serum groups.* New York, NY: Wiley Interscience; 1969. p.390.

Siddiqui B, Hakomori S. *A revised structure for the Forssman glycolipid hapten.* J Biol Chem. 1971; 246: 5766.

Springer GF, Wiener AS. *Alleged causes of the present-day world distribution of the human ABO blood groups.* Nature. 1962; 193: 444.

Springer GF. *T and Tn, general carcinoma autoantigens.* Science. 1984; 224: 1198.

On the Theory of Contingency and Its Relation to Association and Normal Correlation, part of the Research Memoirs Biometric Series I published by the Drapers' Company, 1904.

CHAPTER 14 BLOOD GROUPS AND IMMUNITY, PP. 113–122

Bruce LJ, Beckmann R, Ribeiro ML, Peters LL, Chasis JA, Delaunay J, Mohandas N. Anstee DJ, Tanner MJ. *A band-3 macrocomplex of integral and peripheral proteins in the RBC membrane.* Blood. 2003; 101: 4180.

Chasis JA, Narla M. *Erythroblastic islands: niches for erythropoiesis.* Blood. 2008; 112: 470.

Dahr W, Moulds J. *An immunochemical study on anti-N antibodies from dialysis patients.* Immunol Commun. 1981; 10: 173.

Eyler CE, Telen MJ. *The Lutheran glycoprotein: a multifunctional adhesion receptor.* Transfusion. 2006; 46: 668.

Hadley TJ, Peiper SC. *From malaria to chemokine receptor: The emerging physiologic role of the Duffy blood group antigen.* Blood. 1997; 89: 3077.

Luster AD. *Chemokines: chemotactic cytokines that mediate inflammation.* N Engl J Med. 1998; 338: 436.

Rock JA, Shirey RS, Braine HG, Ness PM, Kickler TS, Niebyl JR. *Plasmapheresis for the treatment of repeated early pregnancy wastage associated with anti-P.* Obstet Gynecol. 1985; 66: 57S.

Spring FA, Parsons SF. *Erythroid call adhesion molecules.* Transfus Med Rev. 2000; 14: 351.

Uchiyama H, Anderson KC. *Cellular adhesion molecules.* Transfus Med Rev. 1994; 8: 84.

CHAPTER 15 THE VALUE OF NULL PHENOTYPES, PP. 123–148

Chrispeels MJ, Agre P. *Aquaporins: Water channel proteins of plant and animal cells.* Trends Biochem Sci. 1994; 19: 421.

Crew VK, Burton N, Kagan A, Green CA, Levene C, Flinter F, Brady L, Daniels G, Anstee DJ. *CD151, the first member of the tetraspanin (TM4) superfamily detected on erythrocytes, is essential for the correct assembly of human basement membranes in kidney and skin.* Blood. 2004; 104: 2217.

Lee S, Russo D, Redman CM. *The Kell blood group system: Kell and XK membrane proteins.* Semin Hematol. 2000; 37: 113.

Mohandas N, Reid ME. *Erythrocyte structure.* In: Young NS, Gerson SL, High KA, editors. *Clinical Hematology.* Philadelphia (PA): Mosby Elsevier; 2006. p.34.

Reid ME. *The Dombrock blood group system: a review.* Transfusion. 2003; 43: 107.

Reid ME, Mohandas N. *Red blood cell blood group antigens: structure and function.* Semin Hematol. 2004; 41: 93.

Reid ME. *The gene encoding the I blood group antigen: review of an I for an eye.* Immunohematology. 2004; 20: 249.

Reid ME, Scientific Publications Committee ABC. *The Rh antigen D: A review for clinicians.* Blood Bulletin. 2008; 10: 1.

Reid ME. *MNS blood group system: a review.* Immunology. 2009; 25: 95.

Sneath JS, Sneath PHA. *Transformation of the Lewis groups of human red cells.* Nature. 1955; 176: 172.

Storry JR, Reid ME. *The Cromer blood group system: a review.* Immunohematology. 2002; 18: 95.

Tippett P, Ellis NA. *The Xg blood group system: A review.* Transfus Med Rev. 1998; 12: 233.

Glossary, pp. 149–162

The American Heritage Dictionary of the English Language, 4th ed. Boston: Houghton Mifflin Company; 2006 .

Epstein AA, Ottenberg R. *Simple method of performing serum reactions.* Proc NY Path Soc. 1908; 8: 117.

Landsteiner K, Wiener AS. *An Agglutinable Factor in Human Blood Recognized by Immune Sera for Rhesus Blood.* Proc Soc Expt Biol Med. 1940; 43: 223-24. In Ottenberg archives at Mt Sinai Hospital library.

Snyder GK, Sheafor BA. *Red blood cells: centerpiece in the evolution of the vertebrate circulatory system.* Amer Zool. 1999; 39: 189.

Soyer A. *The Pantropheon or the History of Food and its Preparation from the earliest ages of the world.* London: Simpkin, Marshall & Co.; 1853. p.287.

General Texts/Sources

Daniels G. *Human blood groups.* 2nd ed. Oxford: Blackwell Scientific Publications; 2002.

Garratty G. editor. *Immunobiology of transfusion medicine.* New York (NY): Marcel Dekker, Inc.; 1994.

Issitt PD, Anstee DJ: *Applied blood group serology.* 4th ed. Durham (NC): Montgomery Scientific Publications; 1998.

Mourant AE, Kopec AC, Domaniewska-Sobczak K. *Distribution of the human blood groups and other polymorphisms.* Vol. 1. 2nd ed. London: Oxford University Press; 1976.

Race RR & Sanger R. *Blood groups in man.* 6th ed. Oxford: Blackwell Scientific Publications; 1975.

Reid ME, Lomas-Francis C. *Blood group antigen FactsBook.* 2nd ed. San Diego

(CA): Academic Press; 2003.

Reid ME, Lomas-Francis C. *Blood group antigens & antibodies: a guide to clinical relevance & technical tips*. New York, (NY): SBB Books. 2007.

SELECTED WEBSITES

For an interactive game about matching ABO groups of donors to patients who were in an accident, see http://nobelprize.org/educational_games/medicine/landsteiner/landsteiner.html

For information about the McLeod syndrome www.nefo.med.uni-muenchen.de/~adanek/McLeod.html

For a website (NHLBI) giving information about blood group alleles with hyperlinks to original scientific reports, enter in a Search Engine "dbRBC". This is quicker and easier than using the full, long address.

Index

FRONTISPIECE and FIG. 1.3: Courtesy of Steven Pierce.

FIG. 1.1: FedEx service marks used by permission.

FIG. 1.2: Courtesy of Yelena Oksov and Gregory Halverson.

FIG. 2.1: © Royal College of Physicians, London.

FIG. 2.2; FIG. 2.3 and FIG. 2.4: © The Royal Society, London.

FIG. 2.5 and FIG. 2.8: Courtesy of the New York Academy of Medicine Library.

FIG. 2.6: The Lionel Pincus and Princess Firyal Map Division, The New York Public Library, Astor, Lenox and Tilden Foundations.

FIG. 2.7 and FIG. 8.5: Courtesy of The South African National Blood Service.

FIG. 2.9: Courtesy of Moir Stamps and Postal History, Australia.

FIG. 3.1; FIG. 6.2; FIG. 6.7; FIG. 8.2 and FIG. 9.2: Courtesy of Patrick Mollison.

FIG. 4.1: © American Medical Woman's Association.

FIG. 6.3 and FIG. 6.4: © Columbia University, College of Physicians and Surgeons.

FIG. 6.5: Based upon Tovey's data presented at the Wellcome symposium, 2003.

FIG. 6.6: Courtesy of Andy Whiteside with permission of Eugene Hamilton's Family.

FIG. 8.1: Courtesy of Robert Coombs.

FIG. 11.1: © Journal of Heredity, courtesy of New York Academy of Medicine.

FIG. 11.2 and FIG. 11.5: Courtesy of The Natural History Museum, New York.

FIG. 11.6: © Anna Shine.

FIG. 15.4: This image was originally published in ASH Image Bank. (2004); John Lazarchick, hereditary elliptocytosis, Fig. 3, 1559-7237 © The American Society of Hematology.

FIG. 15.6: This image was originally published in ASH Image Bank. (2008); Peter Maslak, spherocytes, Fig.1, 1559-7237 © The American Society of Hematology.

FIG. 15.8: This image was originally published in ASH Image Bank. (2009); Peter Maslak, stomatocytes, Fig.1, 1559-7237 © The American Society of Hematology.

FIG. 15.10: This image was originally published in ASH Image Bank. (2005); Peter Maslak, acanthocytosis, Fig.1, 1559-7237 © The American Society of Hematology.

FIG. 15.15: L.H. Bannister, G.H. Michelli, G.A. Butcher, and E.D. Denis: Lamellar membranes associated with rhoptries in erythrocytic merozoites of *Plasmodium knowlesi*: a clue to the mechanism of invasion. *Parasitology* Vol 92, Issue 02, 291-303 (1986). © Cambridge University Press, reproduced with permission.

All other illustrations are by Catherine Hnatov based on diagrams by Marion Reid and Robert Ratner. Cover design by Catherine Hnatov.

We have endeavored to contact all copyright owners. If we have mistakenly missed any copyright holder or given incorrect credit any anyone, we apologize, and request that the copyright owner contact ianshine@verizon.net, and corrections will be made at reprint.

ABOUT THE AUTHORS

Marion Elizabeth Reid, FIMBS, PhD, DSc (Hon.)

Marion Reid was trained as a medical technologist at the North East Metropolitan Blood Transfusion Service, Brentwood, England. She has worked in immunohematology reference laboratories in the UK and USA.

Marion has an extensive serological, biochemical, and molecular knowledge of blood groups and their application to clinical practice and human genetics. Her research has led to the publication of nearly 400 peer-reviewed articles, reviews and chapters. She co-authored *Blood Group Antigens FactsBook*, a well used and respected reference manual for everyday use in the immunohematology laboratories. Marion has served on numerous committees and editorial boards, is a reviewer for several journals, and has received several grants. She is a recognized expert and has been honored by numerous professional awards, including the Ivor Dunsford Award, the Richard Davey Award; the Lyndall Molthan Award; the Bill Teague Award; the Bill Stone Distinguished Speaker Award; the Sally Frank Award; the Council of Hospital Blood Bank Directors Association of Greater New York Award among others.

A much sought-after lecturer, both domestically and internationally, Marion shares her knowledge and experience with different types of audiences-from peers to elementary school children.

Ian Shine, MB, BChir, MD (Cambridge), MD (University of Kentucky)

Trained, University College Hospital. Captain RAMC. Medical Officer, Colonial Service (St. Helena). Scientific Officer, Medical Research Council, Oxford, Post-doctoral Fellow University of Hawaii, Consultant Royal Bucks Hospital, Reading; Assistant Professor, University of Kentucky Medical School; Consultant, Coulter Electronics, Hialeah. Lecturer, Johns Hopkins Medical School.

After running the Thomas Hunt Morgan Institute of Genetics in Lexington for 8 years, he developed a way to measure osmosis that was tested in studies at University College Hospital, London; John Radcliffe Hospital, Oxford; The Royal Society High Altitude Research Laboratory, Interlaken and the Wellcome Laboratories for Comparative Physiology. Many patents (shared with Thomas Shine) have issued.

He published three books and 'A New Strategy to Detect beta-thalassaemia minor' (1970). He found a few new syndromes, and in a patient with carcinoma of the esophagus, presented by Professor Allison at grand rounds in Oxford, he noticed tylosis. It became the second family with the syndrome first reported by Cyril Clarke's team in Liverpool.